Women Come of Age:
Perspectives on the Lives of Older Women

Women Come of Age: Perspectives on the Lives of Older Women

Edited by

Miriam Bernard

and

Kathy Meade

Edward Arnold
A division of Hodder & Stoughton
LONDON MELBOURNE AUCKLAND

© 1993 Miriam Bernard and Kathy Meade

First published in Great Britain 1993

British Library Cataloguing in Publication Data

Bernard, Miriam
  Women Come of Age: Perspectives on the
  Lives of Older Women
  I. Title   II. Meade, Kathy
  305.26
  ISBN 0-340-55261-1

Whilst the advice and information in this book is believed to be true
and accurate at the date of going to press, neither the author nor the
publisher can accept any legal responsibility or liability for any
errors or omissions that may be made.

Typeset in 10/11pt Linotron Times by
Rowland Phototypesetting Limited, Bury St Edmunds, Suffolk.
Printed and bound in Great Britain for Edward Arnold,
a division of Hodder and Stoughton Limited, Mill Road,
Dunton Green, Sevenoaks, Kent TN13 2YA by
Biddles Limited, Guildford and King's Lynn.

Foreword

I do not like writing about being old. This is no doubt partly vanity—we all tend to think of ourselves as perennially young, but partly because society too has such a negative image of what it is like to be old.

But it is also that the subject bores me. I am never conscious of being old, merely of not being able to see very well or take my dogs for as long walks as I used to, or do as much gardening. Otherwise, my life style remains broadly unchanged because it is dominated by the same interests I have had all my life. There are also certain positive advantages. With the ending of the pressures to bring up a family, hold down a job or follow a career one can relax and take time to enjoy the little sensual delights of life like a lovely summer's day. I have learned to live in the moment and worry much less than I used to do.

Of course, I am one of the lucky ones. All my life I have had an interesting, fulfilling and reasonably well rewarded job. It was the one I always wanted—politics—and it was one I could continue on a voluntary basis when I retired professionally. I also enjoy writing and shall continue scribbling until I slip into the grave—probably dictating my own obituary! I am a widow but I have been able to continue to keep my home, one of the centres of our family life.

I am well aware that women on the whole are among the most disadvantaged of our society. It has been my pride and joy to use my political position to help remedy that. The Equal Pay Act, which I got through Parliament in 1970, was far from perfect but it was a break-through, establishing the right to equal pay by law for the first time in our history. That is, of course, only the beginning. We have got to ensure that women get the training for, and access to, the good jobs and the same treatment in pension schemes as received by men. As a Minister I embodied these rights when I introduced the State Earnings Related Pension Scheme.

The moral I draw from all this is that the battle for a happy old age starts quite early in life. I agree with the authors of this book when they write: 'To understand the lives of older women it is necessary to adopt a life-course perspective and to look back at what has gone before'. Later happiness is founded on earlier opportunities and not least on the interests and resources one acquires in youth and this is particularly true for women. Only by working together to win recognition for their rights and abilities all along the line and by taking an interest in the wider world will women be treated as full human beings as they grow older.

I welcome this book as a contribution to this argument.

Barbara Castle

The Right Honourable Baroness of Blackburn
January 1993

Preface
Miriam Bernard and Kathy Meade

Why a book about older women, written by women?

Throughout the 1980s we, the editors, worked with and for older people, mostly in voluntary, research and community development roles and later in higher education and local authority contexts. This experience has made us acutely aware both of what is being done in these areas, but also how little we, our colleagues, our students and the general public appreciate or know about the lives of older people. In our view, such a situation is lamentable. In the UK we are living through an unprecedented time in our history: never before have there been so many old people in the population; and never before has there been such a preponderance of older women.

During the mid-to-late 1980s, our professional paths began to cross more frequently. Although geographically separate (one of us based in London and the other in the Potteries), the community development and research work we were undertaking with Pensioners' Link and The Beth Johnson Foundation brought us into close contact with many older people. In particular, we both became engaged in educational work around health issues (Miriam Bernard, 1985; Kathy Meade, 1986; 1987) and more involved with older women, since they tend to be the overwhelming majority of participants in such activities. With other colleagues, we also worked on the innovative Self Health Care in Old Age Project, training older people to become peer health counsellors and monitoring and evaluating the different elements of this continuing scheme (Miriam Bernard and Vera Ivers, 1986; Bernard, 1988; 1989; Ivers and Meade, 1991). All this helped to sharpen our awareness of the many, and often subtle, ways in which society tends to discriminate against and diminish this sector of the population. In addition, our own lives, influenced by the flourishing of the Women's Liberation Movement in the 1960s and 1970s, alerted us to the process by which women are socialized into positions of subordination and compliance. Every day we saw the cumulative effects of these inequalities as the older women we worked with struggled to maintain their sense of personal and group integrity, while at the same time dealing with the complex effects of the ageing process.

We also found ourselves increasingly frustrated by the paucity of information, research, or even informed discussion, about how women in Britain experience later life. On the international front, initiatives focusing on the situation of older women can be traced back to the early 1980s (see Sheila Peace, 1986, for a history of these developments). Over this decade, important texts appeared on the other side of the Atlantic (Sarah Matthews, 1979; Maxine Szinovacz, 1982; Ellen Gee and Meredith Kimball, 1987; J. Dianne Garner and Susan Mercer, 1989). Over here, in contrast, we had some small-scale pioneering studies undertaken by Helen Evers (1983; 1985) and Alison Froggatt (1985), together with illuminating biographical accounts of women's lives in old age (Susan Hemmings, 1985; Janet Ford and Ruth Sinclair, 1987). 'Ourselves Growing Older'—Jean Shapiro's (1989) self-help guide for women as they age—was also an important contribution and, more recently still, Sara Arber and Jay Ginn (1991c) have usefully examined gender differences in later life.

Despite this, it seemed to us that what we lacked was a holistic review and analysis of what it means to be an older woman living in late twentieth century Britain. Because of our personal histories, professional involvements and intellectual curiosity, we wanted to try to begin to counter the invisibility of older women; to permit their voices to be heard; and their needs and capabilities to be examined in a sensitive and informative way. It was our desire to produce a book in which we could share the information, knowledge and experience both of older women and those working in the broad area of social gerontology.

The book has been written with two particular types of reader in mind. On the one hand, there are a growing number of students within fields such as gerontology, nursing, medicine, social work, social sciences and women's studies, who are increasingly going to want to know more about the circumstances of the women they will be assisting in their professional capacities. For them, we hope this text will provide a stimulating introduction. It should also provide a critical guide to the major issues for the lecturers and researchers associated with these courses. On the other hand, there are those involved in the planning and delivery of services to older adults, who need to understand more fully the social and economic consequences of the ageing process for women. It is our hope that this book will be equally relevant to their concerns. Over and above this, it was also our wish to produce a book written by women, for women, and which women would want to read out of interest, rather than duty! We therefore trust that interested individuals and voluntary groups, as well as academic libraries, will find it accessible and attractive.

The contributors to this book are all women. It was our intention that our experiences as women, working and living out our own lives in a society and in institutions which are clearly and fundamentally still structured through gender, should have a direct bearing on the way in which we approached and developed this book. It was also our explicit desire to work as collectively and cooperatively as possible, despite warnings that this would lead to trouble and interminable delays before the book was published. In the event, we held our first contributors' meeting in London in September 1990, and the final manuscript was with the publishers in August 1992.

In terms of the structure and content of the book, it has been important to us to have a creative tension between the collective nature of the whole enterprise and the individuality of each chapter contributed by our authors. By means of a written brief, through contributors' meetings, and through verbal and written feedback, we have discussed each other's work, made suggestions and amendments to help it all 'hang' together, contributed our ideas and recommendations for the concluding chapter, and agreed the final version.

We are also aware that, in addition to what is as yet a relatively narrow field of academic and popular concern in the UK, there are other limitations to the scope of this book which it is important to share with readers. In particular, we have been conscious from the start that despite our differing origins and ages, and our varied personal and professional backgrounds, we are a group of white, predominantly middle-class women. This means that, to some extent, our own language and circumstances inevitably restrict what we write. Crucially, when we started on this project, we were concerned that there appeared to be no black female gerontologists in this country who might have been able to contribute to this book. However, we were also anxious that issues of race and ethnicity, together with those of class, sexual orientation and disability, were not marginalized into separate chapters, ending up looking like an afterthought. We have thus adopted two means to tackle these difficulties. First, it is our strong conviction that these matters are important dimensions to all the themes covered in this book. Consequently, in our guidelines to contributors we made it clear that, in preparing her chapter, each author needed to address specifically the interests and concerns of these different groups of older women. We also circulated relevant references. Second, in relation to the specific issues affecting the lives of black and minority ethnic older women, we have been fortunate to work in the final production stages with Elaine Arnold, from the University of Sussex. Elaine agreed to read and comment on the manuscript in order to appraise the various points we raise concerning race. This collaboration proved most constructive and helpful to us all.

It will also become increasingly apparent to readers that one notable aspect of this book is the fact that we reference female authors by both their first and second names, at least when they are initially cited in each chapter. Our overriding concern is with the invisibility of women, an invisibility which, like Sue Llewelyn and Kate Osborne (1990), we believe is perpetuated in academic writing and research by the anonymity of using initials. There is an assumption that such work is usually undertaken by men, when this is in fact very far from the truth. For us, it represents one small way by which we are able to reveal women's contribution to our existing body of knowledge.

The process which we have briefly described, and the control which we had over it, was important for us all, as authors and as women. It was also emotional, difficult and stressful at times, as we tried to juggle our commitment to the book with our domestic and professional lives. Of particular value to us was the fact that we were able to share some crucial turning points and transitions which, in microcosm, mirror the developmental perspective we endorse in the book. Our group experienced pregnancies and births, job and career changes, unexpected illnesses and accidents, house moves and long-distance relocations, retirement and bereavement. And, throughout the process of writing, we have all been trying to interweave our roles as women, as writers, as mothers and grandmothers, workers and colleagues, partners, spouses and lovers, and as carers of one kind or another. Above all, it was a challenging, enjoyable and rewarding experience, and one which we hope readers will find equally stimulating.

August 1992

Contents

List of contributors

Miriam Bernard BA, PhD
Is Director of the MA/Diploma and Certificate programmes in Gerontology at the University of Keele. She has researched a wide range of issues relating to older people, and her current interests include leisure; health education and promotion; the needs of carers; pre-retirement education for older women; and evaluation issues and the voluntary sector.

Joanna Bornat BA, PhD
Is a Lecturer at the Open University, in the School of Health, Welfare and Community Education. She is editor of the Journal *Oral History*. She lives in North London and has two grown-up children.

Gillian Dalley BA, MA(Econ), PhD
Gillian Dalley is a senior NHS manager, having previously worked for the Policy Studies Institute and the King's Fund researching health and social security issues. She has three children and lives in London.

Dulcie Groves BA, MSS, PhD
Is an Honorary Lecturer at the University of Lancaster. She retired early, teaches sporadically, researches actively (pensions/women's history), reads widely and enjoys her newfound leisure and travel.

Dorothy Jerrome PhD
Trained as an anthropologist and recently as a counsellor. For many years she was involved in adult education, working with women of all ages. She has undertaken research on women's friendships, associations and experiences of family life.

Kathy Meade BA
Is the Older People's Adviser, Equal Opportunities Unit, London Borough of Hounslow. Her role is to address age discrimination and promote equality of access to council services for older people. She has worked extensively with older people in the community,

particularly around health education, self-help initiatives and pre-retirement preparation.

Sheila M Peace   BA, PhD
Is a Lecturer in the School of Health, Welfare and Community Education at the Open University. Prior to this she was senior research officer and founder member of CESSA (Centre for Environmental and Social Studies on Ageing, University of North London). Since 1975 she has been involved in a wide range of research with older people, particularly in areas of residential care and issues concerning. older women.

Moyra Sidell   BA, SRN, PhD
Is a Research Fellow/Lecturer at the Open University, in the School of Health, Welfare and Community Education. She is currently working on two courses: Health and Well Being, and Death and Dying. Her current research is concerned with health issues and older women. She lives in South London and has grown-up children.

Anthea Tinker   B Com, PhD
Is Director of the Age Concern Institute of Gerontology, University of London and Professor of Social Gerontology, Kings College London. She has undertaken research on older women as carers and on their housing. She has a particular interest in employment and health issues and women's role as grandparents.

Acknowledgements

The development of this book has been a shared enterprise and along the way, numerous people have helped us towards its completion. Our contributors have been supportive throughout: their continuing enthusiasm and involvement in this project has been greatly valued by us both. We would also like to thank Nancy Loffler, our commissioning editor and the six original referees whose constructive and encouraging comments we hope we have encompassed here. Many women's and older people's organizations completed our question-. naire and provided us with valuable details about older women's initiatives throughout the country. In addition we are particularly indebted to Pat, Ray, Joan, Charanjit and Olga who agreed to be interviewed for Chapter 2 and whose photographs grace the front cover.

We would especially like to thank a number of individuals: Elaine Arnold at the University of Sussex for her sensitive and helpful comments on the race dimension; Margaret Bernard for her editorial assistance and her comments on early drafts; and Liesbeth de Block and library staff at the Centre for Policy on Ageing for their help with cross-checking the references.

Thanks go too, to family, friends and colleagues in Stoke, London and New Zealand who have supported, cajoled and humoured us through the ups and downs of the last two years. In addition, our appreciation goes to students on the Gerontology courses at the University of Keele, for their interest and thoughtful responses to some of the material now incorporated in this book.

Lastly, the production of this book and the geographical distance between us has inevitably interfered with our personal lives. Periods of absence, lengthy telephone conversations and the considerable 'overtime' we have put in, is merely the visible evidence of this disruption. Finally then, our special love and gratitude goes to our 'secretaries' and partners—Steve and Mike—for their unwavering practical and emotional support. Together with Mim's small children—Jake and Ben—they have been constant reminders of the need for flexibility and balance in our lives.

Miriam Bernard
Kathy Meade
December 1992

To the older women in our lives who have inspired us and challenged our understanding of what it means to be old and a woman in the 1990s.

1 Perspectives on the lives of older women

Miriam Bernard and Kathy Meade

Introduction

Public, professional and academic interest in ageing is growing rapidly. Yet, it is our belief that the experiences of older people in general, and older women in particular, are very often misrepresented and undervalued. Not only are lay and professional perceptions largely negative, but academic research, and particularly policy-oriented research, has tended to reinforce this view, being focused largely on a problem-oriented notion of old age in modern society (Bond and Coleman, 1990; Sara Arber and Jay Ginn, 1991b). Given that women form the vast majority of the older population— there are now nearly seven million women over the age of 60—then it is evident that they will experience these disadvantages more often, and indeed for longer, than older men. In later life, the impact of the very different life-course experiences of men and women do not, to use Sheila Peace's (1986) phrase, 'magically disappear'. Rather, women also feel the complex and compound effects of patriarchy and structural disadvantage in old age.

In this book, we concentrate on older women in the UK. We try to look at older women 'in the round', examining their current situations and exploring how they contend with the various demands and pressures upon them. Our aim is not to minimize the very real problems many of us face as we age, but to analyse the underlying reasons for them and to perhaps provide different visions of what old age might hold for women. Due to the lack of research literature and of experience drawn from practice, we are attempting to map out our current state of knowledge and, in the process, probably raise as many questions as answers.

A number of key concerns and issues have informed the construction of the whole book. First, we argue, as others have done before us (Bond *et al.*, 1990; Ellen Gee and Meredith Kimball, 1987), that the study of ageing and of older women should be a multidisciplinary undertaking. Indeed, our own backgrounds reflect this. Second, as a group of women writing about women, our desire was to work within a consensus that we felt would enable us to make sense of the variety of experiences that women both bring to, and contend with in, old age. Thus, our writings are influenced by a shared belief that it is the structures, policies and ideology of western capitalist society that are a major cause of women's relative social and economic powerlessness. In societies such as ours that are systematically, as well as dramatically and graphically, at times sexist, racist and ageist in turn, then it is hardly surprising that amongst the myriad disadvantaged groups older women feature particularly strongly. Third, we all share a conviction that it is important to understand women's lives from a life-course perspective, and from what may be broadly described as a feminist viewpoint. These perspectives, together with increasing age consciousness within our society, and a related and growing concern with what has been misleadingly heralded as the 'demographic timebomb', are the issues we take up in this opening chapter, providing the reader with a framework in which to set the succeeding contributions.

Older women and demographic change

In late twentieth century Britain ageing is very much an issue for, and about, women. Discussions of the underlying causes of population ageing, together with detailed statistics, can be found in a number of recent texts and fact sheets and in regular publications from the Office of Population Censuses and Surveys (OPCS) and the Central Statistical Office (CSO, 1989; OPCS, 1989a; Arber and Ginn, 1991c; Christina Victor, 1991; Wells and Freer, 1988; Age Concern Institute of Gerontology, 1991; Family Policy Studies Centre, 1991; Anthea Tinker, 1992). Our intention here is to describe what is distinctive about the demography of older women and to draw out some of the key features.

At the turn of the century just under two million people were of pensionable age; we now have in the region of ten and a half million elderly people in the UK, representing a fivefold increase. Of these, some two-thirds are women. This numerical imbalance between the sexes becomes more pronounced with increasing age. Older women are survivors; they account for 58 per cent of people over the age of 60, 67 per cent of people over the age of 75, and 80 per cent of those surviving to 90 or older.

Two of the major contributory factors are reductions in mortality and differing increases in life expectancy since the turn of the century: then, life expectancy at birth was only about 50 years; currently it is in the region of 79 years for women and 73 years for men. When we compare the life expectancy of older people today with older people then, we find that although it has increased less dramatically, a woman who is aged 65 today can expect to live for just over 17 more years as opposed to 12, and a man of the same age for approximately 13 more years as opposed to 11 (OPCS, 1989b). This faster reduction in female mortality has resulted in what is now termed 'the feminization of later life' (Arber and Ginn, 1991c). Mortality rates at younger ages have been considerably reduced and death, which used to be a marked feature of early childhood, is now an expectation of old age. Indeed, for many women it is an expectation of great old age (Mike Bury and Anthea Holme, 1991). In addition, over the same time period we have witnessed a dramatic fall in the birth rate. Today, the average family size in the UK fluctuates around, or just below, replacement level: this, in combination with decreased mortality at all ages, has produced our ageing population.

Because of these rapid changes in mortality and fertility, current cohorts of older women are now in a unique position: in many instances they are members of families which are top-heavy with adults (Dorothy Jerrome, 1990a). Indeed, it is now possible to be both a grandmother and a granddaughter simultaneously. In addition, the demographic imbalance between the sexes is further reflected in distinct differences in marital status and living arrangements. While the propensity to marry has become almost universal, a greater proportion of men will still be married in old age. Women's greater life expectancy dictates that they will probably outlive their partners and, indeed, over the age of 65 only 38 per cent of women are married compared with 73 per cent of men (OPCS, 1990b).

The converse of this is that a substantial proportion of women are widows in old age: over the age of 65, 50 per cent of women are widowed, compared with only 17 per cent of men (OPCS, 1990b). And, as women grow older, widowhood increases; rising to nearly two-thirds of those over the age of 75, and three-quarters of those aged 85 and over. Consequently, widowhood is the likely condition that the majority of married women will face in later life. There is also a large number of older women who, by choice or by force of circumstance, have never married. With the increase in the rate of marriage noted above, remaining 'single' will, in theory at least, become much less common (Emily Grundy, 1983). However, these categories for marital status may not continue to reflect the reality of living arrangements. For example, a childless woman who was briefly married may be more analogous to the 'traditional' single woman than either a technically never-married older woman with a partner and children, or lesbian couples.

What we are also seeing, in most western societies, is a rising divorce rate. At present, under 5 per cent of older people are divorced, but this is expected to increase dramatically as higher numbers enter old age with at least one divorce behind them. On current trends, it has been estimated that by 2025 one in eight women aged 65 and over will be divorced, compared with one in thirty-nine in 1990 (Family Policy Studies Centre, 1991). Marriage itself is still popular and, despite the probable outcome, the majority of divorced people will marry again. With increasing age however, we find that divorced and widowed women are much less likely to remarry than their male counterparts (OPCS, 1990d). Part of the explanation for this obviously lies in women's greater longevity, but research also suggests that marriage, whilst advantageous for men's mental health and wellbeing, is less satisfying for women (Jessie Bernard, 1976; Mildred Blaxter, 1990). In Helena Lopata's (1973) classic study of widows for example, only one-fifth expressed a desire to remarry. Even if older women do not directly experience divorce and remarriage themselves, it is still likely to affect their lives. The dividing and blending of existing partnerships will have particular implications for their relationships with children and grandchildren, for their financial and housing situations, for their own health, and for their access to caring and other resources in old age.

Marital status is also closely reflected in patterns of household formation and living arrangements. The number of older people living alone today is historically unprecedented (Angela Dale *et al.*, 1987) and, given the many widows, it comes as no surprise to find almost half of women over the age of 65 in this situation. Gender differences in marital status mean that older women, and particularly very old women, will be much more likely to spend their last years in institutional settings. Indeed, Arber and Ginn (1991c) note that it is 'those "closest" to marriage and children (who) are least likely to enter a residential establishment' (p.154).

Finally, in considering these demographic issues, we are conscious that the general trends we are describing obscure other distinctions we might wish to make. For example, life expectancy, birth and mortality rates will differ according to both where, and in what circumstances one lives, and to which racial or ethnic group one belongs (Townsend *et al.*, 1988; OPCS, 1990d). In the UK we are only just beginning to recognize and acknowledge the ethnic dimensions to ageing, despite a history which dates back at least to Roman times (Fryer, 1984). As Maggie Pearson (1991) maintains, it is also still the case that: 'If black and ethnic minority communities have been "invisible" in Britain, their elders have been all the more so' (p.437).

Recent figures (Haskey, 1990) suggest that there are almost half a million people of pensionable age living here who were born abroad, representing about 5 per cent of the entire elderly population. Of these, the largest proportions are of Afro-Caribbean and Asian extraction; smaller numbers originate from Poland and from other EC and Eastern European countries, from Ireland, and from China and East Asia. The geographical distribution of these groups is very unbalanced, with concentrations in certain urban and inner city areas. While there are a growing number of empirical studies concerning the personal, health, social and economic situations of black and minority ethnic older people, much of it is of a piecemeal and fragmented nature (Amanda Squires, 1991; Barker, 1984b; Berry *et al.*, 1981; Bhalla and Blakemore, 1981; Marian Farrah, 1986; Fenton, 1986; Glendenning and Pearson, 1988; Alison Norman, 1985). Instead, what we do have are 'a number of potent stereotypes about the "more caring" nature of minority communities' (Victor, 1991, p.34): stereotypes which, given that women take on the bulk of these responsibilities (see p.113), have particular ramifications for the situations of older women. More gender-differentiated work in this key area is, we feel, urgently needed because, as Christina Victor (1991) notes: 'A feature of British society in the next 25 years will be the ageing of the ethnic minority communities who came to the country in the 1960s' (p.33). Our response should be now, and it has to be flexible and sensitive to the varied interests and needs of these groups (Pearson, 1991; Bond and Coleman, 1990).

We need also to consider some of the various perspectives concerning this issue; both those that have been, and those that might be, used to study women's lives in old age. In this book we concentrate on three broad areas: feminist, social gerontological and life-course perspectives. While each of these approaches brings with it a certain body of theoretical and methodological knowledge, it is our contention that their potential for informing our understanding of the lives of older women has yet to be fully realized.

Older women: specifying what we mean

Definitions of old age have varied throughout history and in different cultural and social circumstances. During this century we have seen various attempts to define old age in relation to straight chronology, linked with significant life events such as retirement from paid work and, latterly, in terms of functional or 'status' constructions (Midwinter, 1991a; Laslett, 1989). Although there is little consensus over the 'best' or most appropriate way of defining old age, we need to acknowledge that, during a period which may span 30 years or more, it is likely that different definitions will be more or less suitable at different times.

Despite this, chronological age is still a popular way of differentiating phases of the life course, and of segregating people. The onset of old age is usually regarded as synonymous with the statutory retirement age which, for women, means that reaching 60 years of age heralds the beginning of this phase. A notable development of the mid 1970s was the tendency to begin to divide older people into two age categories. The eminent American gerontologist Bernice Neugarten (1974; 1975) was one of the first to propose such a division, labelling people aged 55 to 74 years of age as 'young–old' and those over the age of 75 as 'old–old'. In this country however, the lower age boundary was more often set at age 65 as opposed to 55 (Abrams, 1978; 1980; Audrey Hunt, 1978). More recently, people over the age of 85 have been defined as the 'oldest–old' or the 'very elderly' (Binstock, 1985). However, what seems to have been forgotten is that these distinctions were originally made on the basis of health status (Arber and Ginn, 1991c), whereas nowadays they are often used uncritically as convenient administrative cutoff points. Subdividing old people into ever smaller age categories also hinders our analysis of the wide variations in other characteristics they may exhibit.

Growing dissatisfaction with chronological definitions has led to an emphasis on functional definitions and status constructs which are based on position in the social life cycle (Midwinter, 1991a). In the latter case, the life course is divided into four ages: the First Age of childhood and socialization; the Second Age of paid work and family raising; the Third Age of active independent life beyond work and parenting; and the Fourth Age of eventual dependence. Definitions such as these go some way towards counteracting the negative connotations of our changing demography. For example, there is growing evidence that the Third Age in particular can be a time of renewed interest in cultural and educational activities (Featherstone, 1987; Laslett, 1989; Schuller and Young, 1991). However, we need to temper this enthusiasm somewhat and question whether the 'active independent life' of the Third Age is really within the reach of the majority of older women. This is one of the particular themes we develop through this book as we explore whether older women have the means—economic, social or cultural—to make this a reality. Furthermore, constructing the Fourth Age as a period of dependence still confines older people to a passive, powerless and unfortunate situation.

We do however concur with Eric Midwinter (1991a) when he argues that 'birthdays are poor indicators of social attitudes or health factors' (p.6). For women these two issues are extremely important, for the negative social attitudes which pervade our society are commonly linked with the expectation that old age brings declining health. This is explored further in the chapter by Moyra Sidell, but here it is worth noting that measures of functional disability are particularly significant in highlighting gender differentials in old age (Arber and Ginn, 1991c). Such definitions also have implications for the help that older women might require. It may be, for example, that in the current drive towards community care, functional definitions will be most useful for those professionals charged with arranging and managing care packages for older women. Chronological age alone, we must stress, bears no simple or direct relation to levels of disability or functioning.

We want the reader to be clear about how we are using the term 'older women'. For the sake of simplicity we shall, in the main, be regarding women over the age of 60 as 'old'. Where appropriate, our contributors make various distinctions within this group according to functional ability, social status, class and race. In thinking about the future, it is also important to consider the generations of women who are now middle-aged; our contributors at times refer to women who may currently be in their fifties. Finally, whilst 'older women' is our preferred term, readers need to be aware that we sometimes use this interchangeably with the phrase 'elderly women'.

Older women and the life course

It is our view that the life course provides one particularly useful framework within which to study human development and behaviour. As contributors to this book, we are all interested in understanding the emotional and psychological contexts in which women age, as well as concerned with how these interact with the more socially constructed factors discussed later in this chapter. We examine how some authors have studied human ageing as a logical extension of developmental psychology, and argue that many of the traditional models and theories do not take full account of older women's experiences. The growing interest in what is now termed life-span developmental psychology may provide a much needed corrective, and enable us to study more accurately the psychology of ageing from a female perspective.

It is clear that using age-banded stages or phases is one way in which psychologists concerned with human development have traditionally divided up the life course. Until comparatively recently developmental psychologists paid little attention to the phases beyond the First Age of childhood and adolescence. We can identify a number of key issues which underlie this neglect of adult development, of the lives of older people in general, and of the experiences of older women in particular.

First, the notion that we can divide up the life course into rigid stages, often marked by particular chronological ages (Havighurst, 1953), derives from a very specific biological concept of development. The human organism is seen as following a linear process of maturation and decline (Charlotte Buhler, 1935; Lidz, 1976). This process is marked by its universality, in which we all follow a given route towards some end state. To reach this end state, we must successfully negotiate each stage before passing onto the next. In each stage we are also supposed to take on particular roles or statuses such as marriage or the formation of a family; not to do so is somehow deviant. Such a view seems to us to be very inflexible and deterministic. It fails to acknowledge the ebb and flow of life, and hinders our understanding of the different paths that individual development might take. Crucially too, it minimizes the influence of the social environment on human development (Marjorie Fiske and David Chiriboga, 1985).

Second, a great deal of emphasis has been placed on the early, formative stages of the life course. Peter Coleman (1990a) has noted the suspicion and reluctance of British psychologists to include adult life under the rubric of developmental psychology. He also observes that the British Society of Developmental Psychology is explicitly. devoted to child development. No wonder then that the popular view of human development is that it seems to cease at about the age of 21! Even with the growth of studies on adult development, Sue Llewelyn and Kate Osborne (1990) have recently remarked that:

'Although an enormous amount has been written about the first half of the life span, until very recently it seems as if there has been a conspiracy of silence about growing older, suggesting a widespread view of the second half of life that is somehow less valuable or important than the first half' (p.226).

A third difficulty we are faced with is that many stage theories take very little account of social, environmental or cultural contexts and, therefore, the marked differences in both the private and public arenas in which people live out their lives. A simple example of this is the substantial number of women, now in their eighties, who have remained single because the loss of men in the First World War severely reduced their chances of marrying (Margot Jefferys and Pat Thane, 1989). Far from being deviant, their civil status has been socially constructed, a fact which is not understood by those who make derogatory comments about 'old spinsters'.

Fourth, psychological research in general, and developmental psychology is no exception to this, has tended to ignore women and neglect women's issues (Susan Gaylord, 1989). For example, Erik Erikson's (1950) classic work focuses on the eight 'ages of man', while more recent explorations also concentrate on male subjects (Levinson *et al.*, 1978). As yet, we have insufficient empirical research to assess whether or not these theories are equally applicable to women. Writers have responded in varying ways to this challenge. Erikson's later work on old age (Erikson *et al.*, 1986) has concentrated on developing the notion of 'ego integrity': the task of finding meaning and order in one's life, and accepting it for what it is. He and his colleagues point out some of the key areas of adjustment for older people that are of equal importance for both women and men.

Other psychologists have responded by formulating separate theories of women's identity development (Carol Gilligan, 1982; Carol Franz and Kathleen White, 1985). This should help us counter the notion that women somehow reflect an incomplete and inferior development when judged against male-orientated developmental standards (Leonie Sugarman, 1986).

We therefore have to ask some hard questions about the applicability of such models and theories to the lives of women, and in particular to the lives of older women. There now exists a steadily growing appreciation of the fact that we cannot consider old age in isolation from what has gone before. This holistic view or, as Leonie Sugarman (1986) describes it, 'a total-life-span, total-life-space approach to human development' (p.24), is at the heart of the revival of interest in life-span developmental psychology. Advocates of this approach subscribe to a general perspective which is concerned with 'a changing individual in a changing society' (Sugarman, 1986, p.46). Although as yet it has had relatively little influence on the study of ageing in general, proponents believe it provides a fruitful context for the study of the psychology of ageing (Coleman, 1990a). It is our contention that such an approach is crucial to our understanding of the situations which confront women as they age. Life-span developmental psychology emphasizes the importance of individual history; it recognizes that development occurs on different fronts and at variable rates; and it acknowledges the interaction of the individual with the environment (Sugarman, 1986). This captures the essence of the orientation we adopt in this book, for it suggests that, as individuals, we have the psychological capacity for continued change, both in relation to our own personality and capabilities, and in respect of our interrelationships with other people and with society in general. Finally, it is an approach which does not write women off just because of their particular age, class, race or sexual orientation.

Perspectives from social gerontology

Social gerontology is an eclectic discipline, and borrows freely from a number of different perspectives. Here, we concentrate on approaches drawn mainly from sociology in order to review what they have to say about the experience of growing older. Detailed discussions of the main theoretical orientations can be found in Dianne Garner and Susan Mercer (1989), Gee and Kimball (1987) and Fennell *et al.* (1988). For now, we shall briefly examine role and activity theory; disengagement theory; continuity theory; exchange theory; and the political economy perspective.

The first three theories are couched within the structural–functionalist perspective in sociology and, more specifically, within a consensual view of how society functions. In the words of Susan McDaniel (1989), this is a view which: 'focuses on social order premised on cooperation, interdependence, and shared values, adjustment by the individual to society, and societal equilibrium' (p.52). In relation to older people, it tends to reinforce the belief that they represent a major social problem, and led to extensive theorizing from the 1950s onwards about how individuals best adjust to old age. Role and activity theory, and disengagement theory are the most well-known versions of this perspective.

Role theory, which became popular in the 1950s, argues that individual behaviour is largely determined by the social roles we perform. Not surprisingly, the key social role is that of worker and, in a society organized around the work ethic, the loss of work upon retirement is regarded as particularly harmful to one's self-esteem and morale. These arguments were revised with the appearance of disengagement theory in the early 1960s (Elaine Cumming and William Henry, 1961). This theory contends that, as part of normal ageing, there is a mutual withdrawal between the individual and others in society. This process may be initiated by oneself, or by other people, but it is regarded as both natural and inevitable. Over time, the individual becomes increasingly self-absorbed in preparation for death. Again, maintenance of morale is key and, in this theory, is positively associated with disengagement. For men, disengagement is commonly marked by retirement from paid employment. For women, widowhood was conventionally seen as the formal start of this process.

Both role theory and disengagement theory were developed largely in relation to the working man and, in particular, in connection with formal retirement from paid work. If women were considered at all, it was simply to argue that retirement was in fact much less psychologically wounding because of the 'other' roles they maintain. Disengagement too was regarded as easier for women, as they do not experience the major upheavals accompanying men's retirement. However, even where women are not in paid work, old age brings with it the loss of other roles. Like men, older women may also be faced with trying to find new roles and activities. In addition, disengagement theory has been roundly criticized for overlooking the fact that it may well be involuntary and take place, if at all, in different ways and at different rates for men and women (McDaniel, 1989). Nor is it necessarily inevitable or desirable. Indeed, it may be one way in which society is able to sanction its disinterest in the real difficulties and problems many people face throughout old age (Ethel Shanas *et al.*, 1965).

As a counter to these theories, activity theory emphasizes the means by which psychological and social wellbeing can be maintained in old age through involvement in new activities. Much literature now exists extolling the virtues of an active retirement, and the once popular notion of 'successful ageing' is itself premised on the desirability of maintaining a variety of interests in old age (Havighurst, 1963). This theory too has been criticized, both for its idealistic nature (Bond *et al.*, 1990) and for the new and often unrealistic set of pressures it may put on older people. The stereotype of the ever-active granny is just as hard to shake off as its miserable and disengaged counterpart!

These theories focus predominantly on the individual and, in research terms, have concentrated on issues such as wellbeing; adjustment to ageing; and role changes and transitions. Whereas role and disengagement theory emphasize the discontinuities in people's lives, later theories highlight the continuous threads which run through our entire biographies. Continuity theory looked initially at work histories and work careers, with research in the 1960s within this framework concentrating very much on adjustment to retirement. It was argued that if social involvement and favourable self-esteem—both of which were seen as being anchored in work—were not established before retirement, then they were unlikely to be created afterwards (Fennell *et al.*, 1988).

Again, women were largely left out of this discussion, at least until later empirical studies. Sarah Matthews' research (1979; 1986) for example, looks at how older women maintain a positive identity in the face of the stigmatizing experiences of daily life. One way is through the continuities they have in terms of relationships and activities, together with their identification with what Matthews (1979) calls a 'setting', be it the home or local neighbourhood. As Graham Fennell and his colleagues (1988) contend:

'Such continuities are not uniquely important to women, of course, but they are perhaps especially important in women's lives, given the powerful negative stereotypes which apply particularly to them (and to which they themselves may subscribe) and given also the structured disadvantages of old women with respect to income and other resources' (pp.105–6).

Sarah Matthews' work was greatly influenced by symbolic–interactionist perspectives in sociology and social psychology. Here, the emphasis was on trying to understand how individuals interpret and give meaning to their actions (Bond *et al.*, 1990). These ideas are also at the core of social exchange theory which: 'in a somewhat different vein, looks at how older people deal with diminished resources in their exchange relationships with other people' (Gee and Kimball, 1987, p.7).

Traditionally, exchange theory was again rooted in the notion of work in the sense that one 'exchanged' one's labour for financial remuneration. Interaction between groups and individuals was sustained only for as long as it was 'profitable'. For the present cohorts of older women, workforce participation has often been secondary to family roles, with the result that their 'resources' are usually not of the financial kind (see p.49). For them, exchanges have, and still do, take place within the context of family relationships (Janet Finch, 1989). There are however difficulties in using exchange theory as a basis for understanding social relationships since, as Argyle and Henderson (1984) argue, people often cannot end a relationship even when they appear to get nothing from it. Moreover, much of it was premised on a belief that older people became less and less able to reciprocate, to the extent that the only currency they could bring to the exchange was esteem built up in the past and compliance with whatever might be on offer (Dowd, 1980). We are dealing here, as Phillipson and Walker (1987) argue, with a damaging ideology and view of old age which holds up the spectre of a society composed increasingly of old, sick, dependent and poor people. In a differing guise, exchange theory has helped fuel the renewed and pernicious debate concerning the potential for intergenerational conflict over scarce resources (Johnson *et al.*, 1989; Phillipson, 1991; Thomson, 1989).

Arising out of these theories, the 1970s and 1980s witnessed the growth of what has become known as the political economy perspective. In the UK, the work of Peter Townsend, Alan Walker and Chris Phillipson has been particularly influential in developing this critical, as opposed to purely descriptive, approach to the study of old age (Townsend, 1981; 1986; Walker, 1981; 1982; Phillipson, 1982; Phillipson and Walker, 1986; 1987). This view is primarily concerned with how economic and political factors, such as retirement and pensions policies, restrict older people's access to a wide range of resources. Importantly, it analyses the inequalities which exist in the distribution of these resources, not from an individual point of view, but in relation to the distribution of power within society (Arber and Ginn, 1991c; Kart, 1987).

A political economy perspective is potentially of great significance in understanding women's lives in old age. Yet, writers on this side of the Atlantic have, as Sara Arber and Jay Ginn (1991b) state, concentrated largely on class as the main way of stratifying their analyses. Gender-differentiated work within this perspective is limited. It poses difficulties, not least because there is no acceptable or agreeable way (as yet) of assigning social classes to older women. Usually, this is based on their spouse's last or current occupation or, in the case of single women, on their own last occupation. Ageing, however, is a gendered process, and 'growing old and female may be very different from growing old and male' (Gee and Kimball, 1987, p.8). Although the political economy perspective has begun to raise critical questions concerning how women experience growing old within our patriarchal society, we still need to extend this and develop theoretical and analytical frameworks which take full account of the fact that the study of old age is very much a woman's issue.

Feminism and older women

One response to the invisibility of women has been the development of feminism. However, with some notable exceptions (Barbara Mac-Donald and Cynthia Rich, 1984; Meg Stacey, 1989; Zelda Curtis, 1989) feminism has yet to really address the central issues with which we are concerned here; namely, understanding and illuminating the lives of older women. Below, we explore some of the reasons for this neglect, but first it is important to preface what we have to say with a short description of the major perspectives that the term 'feminism' encompasses.

Feminism is a broad philosophical framework concerned with issues around equality, empowerment and social change for both men and women (Karla Henderson *et al.*, 1989). The historical development of contemporary feminism as a political movement has been discussed by numerous writers (Anna Coote and Bea Campbell, 1982; Hester Eisenstein, 1984; Anne Phillips, 1987; Juliet Mitchell and Ann Oakley, 1986; Caroline Ramazanoglu, 1989; Rosemarie Tong, 1989). Helen Crowley and Susan Himmelweit (1992) have also argued that this has been paralleled at every stage by a complementary academic interest. No single feminist perspective exists, and in recent years different authors have suggested a wide variety of classifications. Rosemarie Tong (1989) identifies seven categories: liberal; socialist; radical; Marxist; existentialist; psychoanalytic; and postmodern. Bea Campbell (1987) raises the issue of whether or not we can include, as feminists, some of the women who are active in the Conservative Party. Linda McDowell and Rosemary Pringle (1992) remind us that there are other possible categories of feminism based on issues such as sexual orientation or race. Typically though, three broad approaches can be identified: liberal feminism; socialist feminism; and radical feminism.

Differences between these approaches centre around philosophical, methodological and political concerns, and these may at times conflict with each other (Shulamit Reinharz, 1989). However, according to a number of writers all forms of feminism share some common assumptions and goals (Liz Stanley and Sue Wise, 1983; Henderson *et al.*, 1989; Crowley and Himmelweit, 1992): all are concerned with improving the lot of women through individual and societal change; with making visible their experiences; with achieving equality, dignity and freedom of choice; and with removing all forms of inequity and oppression in society. Where these perspectives differ importantly one from another is in the means they put forward to achieve change.

Liberal feminism's central concern is with discrimination against women, believing that change will be brought about through strategies such as legislation and practical help to assist women who want to combine careers with family life. This emphasis on ensuring that the rights of individuals are safeguarded does not challenge the fundamental beliefs of society. Rather, it places the major emphasis on the individual's private life, arguing that women should be integrated into the existing structures by means of equality of opportunity and equal access (Henderson *et al.*, 1989). Described by Alice Rossi (1969) as 'the feminist-assimilation model', it has been criticized on the grounds that liberal solutions only improve the lot of some women, and that they are based on the false assumption that our existing white, and male-dominated, social structures represent an ideal society.

Radical and socialist feminists, by contrast, take a structural view of women's subordination, and argue for fundamental changes in the way our society is organized. Socialist feminists suggest that through the process of sex-role socialization, women have become locked into a subordinate and oppressed position. It is only by examining the societal causes of this oppression, causes which are also closely tied to the exploitation suffered by the working classes, and by transforming the institutions that make up this oppressive structure, that women's position will change.

Radical feminism takes a somewhat different stance in that it regards women, not society, as the central issue. Adopting the slogan 'the personal is political', its proponents set about challenging the belief that women are only of importance or consequence when defined in relation to men. They promote women's self-determination and autonomy, arguing that women need to be at the hub of any new social order (Henderson *et al.*, 1989).

In the context of this book, we adopt Shulamit Reinharz's (1989) position that 'feminism will be defined as their sum' (p.25). Moreover, feminism is currently trying to grapple with postmodernist ideas, which return us to the core historical debates around equality or difference which have characterized feminist thought over the years (McDowell and Pringle, 1992). These issues impose a requirement on us, as contributors to this book, both to recognize and examine the similarities which exist, and to acknowledge and make explicit the fact that older women, like all women, are divided by class, age, sexual orientation, race, ethnic origin and other factors.

Given that one of the unique characteristics of feminism has, up until now, been its woman-centredness, one might have expected that the issues affecting older women would have played a crucial part in its historical development. However, much feminist research and writing to date has reflected what can only be described as the ageism of the women's movement itself. In America, Shulamit Reinharz (1989) has noted that since about 1970, each feminist perspective has been developing analyses of ageing, but here in the UK, Sara Arber and Jay Ginn (1991c) have recently contended that ageing has not been part of the feminist agenda. In this country younger feminists have seldom raised or discussed issues and problems specific to older women (Curtis, 1989): a situation which has led Susan Hemmings (1985) to comment on the Women's Liberation Movement in these terms:

> 'Any woman older than.this (about 45) within the movement has been treated there much as she is outside it: as cranky, boring, bossy, neurotic, and politically backward. There is a kind of tension in groups when she speaks in case she wanders off the point, or says something outrageously reactionary' (p.5).

Some of the reasons for the neglect of older women are themselves historical, in that twenty years ago or more priorities and issues were different. Then, feminists who were themselves young were primarily interested in issues of importance to younger women, such as childcare, reproduction and inequalities in labour market participation. Life beyond the menopause seemed insignificant by comparison. These issues have dominated feminist agendas, not least because feminist researchers have tended to research their own current concerns. Methodologically and philosophically however, feminist research is of great relevance in our quest to understand better the lives of older women. And, as feminists themselves age, we might postulate that research about ageing and about issues of importance to older women are likely to come more to the fore; a book about women, ageing and the menopause by Germaine Greer (1991), entitled 'The Change', being but one recent example.

For feminists, it was issues of class and race which first triggered an examination of the differences which exist among women. During the last decade too, some feminists have begun to turn their attention, if not explicitly towards the ageing process, at least towards older women. Unfortunately however, this has been a very selective enterprise, tending to focus almost exclusively on caring and community care policies. In one sense, this comes as no surprise, given that over the last twenty years or so, the concept of 'care in and by the community' has become a linchpin of government social policy. As Isobel Allen (1988) contends, it is this interest, shown by governments of whatever political persuasion, that has at last prompted feminists 'to wake up to the fact that ageing might be a feminist issue' (p.36).

In their work, feminists have drawn links between the care of older people and the care of young children, challenging the assumptions underlying community care policies that, it is forcefully argued, rely on the willingness and availability of family members, i.e. women, to provide such services for dependant relatives (Gillian Dalley, 1988; Clare Ungerson, 1987). Feminists have also successfully striven to make visible the sacrifices and hardships involved in caring; highlighting the emotional, psychological, social and economic costs entailed with such activity (Jenny Pulling, 1987; Jill Pitkeathley, 1989). A key aim has been to lift caring out of the privacy and obscurity of the domestic setting and to describe it as labour (Janet Finch and Dulcie Groves, 1983; Muriel Nissel and Lucy Bonnerjea, 1982), worthy at least of recognition and, ideally, of financial remuneration (Kari Waerness, 1990).

Without minimizing the importance of this work it may, unwittingly, have helped contribute to what Arber and Ginn (1991b) describe as 'a pathological view of elderly people' (p.261). In the first place, early research on caring tended to concentrate very much on the carers. One reason for this was that the feminist campaign to extend the 1975 Invalid Care Allowance to married women required unequivocal evidence of the demands being made on them as frontline carers (see pp.120–23). This inevitably meant that the experiences and reactions of those being cared for received minimal attention, despite the attempts of some researchers (Finch and Groves, 1982; Finch, 1984). The overall result has been a very one-dimensional picture, in which elderly people are stereotyped as the passive recipients of care.

Second, and again unsurprisingly, such research was primarily concerned with women as carers and, more particularly, with daughters as carers. This has also helped to stereotype our view of them as middle-aged women 'caught in the middle' (Elaine Brody, 1981) between their obligations to children and to elderly dependants. The inaccuracy of this view has begun to be widely challenged in the last few years, highlighting the contributions of elderly people themselves, and of men, to the caring process (see pp.110–13).

A third challenge to this strand of feminist writing has come from the disability movement. They attack the perception and treatment of disabled women as somehow different from other women; for assuming that caring is always burdensome, and for perpetuating the belief that disabled women cannot also be carers (Jenny Morris, 1991).

Researching older women

Although one might justifiably criticize feminist research, it is important in both conceptual and methodological terms. Conceptually, feminist research begins from the basis that all women are oppressed, and has at its core the aims of examining the shared features of that experience; making visible the lives of women; of giving them a voice; and of articulating the positive contributions that women make. Methodologically, it espouses the view that research cannot be a value-free undertaking, and that its outcomes are affected by the researcher herself: a role which should be both acknowledged and utilized. Using qualitative approaches in which women interview women, establishing trust and sensitively uncovering and understanding the experiences described by respondents are also key (Oakley, 1981).

These developments parallel the increasing emphasis, in gerontological circles, on the use of life history or biographical approaches (Joanna Bornat, 1989; Johnson, 1978; Peace, 1990). A decade ago, Helen Evers (1983) endorsed the value of a life-course approach in her study of women aged 75 years and over, while Malcolm Johnson (amongst others) has long argued the benefits of biographical studies in work with older people. More recently, Fennell *et al.* (1988) analyse the usefulness of these kinds of approaches, arguing that although such methods have 'hitherto been longer on advocacy than on the production of results' (p.78), they do have the potential to advance our knowledge and understanding.

The work of Susan Hemmings (1985), of Janet Ford and Ruth Sinclair (1987) and of Suzanne Nield and Rosalind Pearson (1992) are examples of the powerful ways in which biographical and qualitative approaches can illuminate both individual lives and social history. These books contain transcripts of conversations with middle-aged and older women and, whilst many describe their difficulties in adjusting to old age, they also display considerable courage and resourcefulness in the face of adversity. Teasing out the intricacies of daily lives and past experiences in this way helps us to understand more fully the choices and constraints (both individually and socially constructed) under which we all attempt to fashion our current lifestyles.

In tandem with this work, we would also argue that all forms of social research with older people need to be gender-sensitive as a matter of course. There are some notable examples of existing longitudinal studies which have attempted to look, for instance, at gender and social class inequalities, at the kinds of resources which promote wellbeing in later life (Taylor and Ford, 1983; Taylor, 1988), or more generally at the lives of older women (Insa Fooken, 1985). It would also be useful, in our view, to have comprehensive gender-based (re-)analyses of large data sets such as the General Household Survey (GHS), together with concerted efforts to triangulate evidence from different sources (Leonie Kellaher *et al.*, 1990).

More recently too, feminist researchers have been concerned to explore ways to enable women, as the traditional 'objects' or 'subjects' of research, to have a more active and empowering role in the research process (Sherna Berger Gluck and Daphne Patai, 1991; Helen Roberts, 1992). Yet, although feminist research has undoubtedly corrected some of the inadequacies in traditional, male-dominated research processes and methodologies, it still needs to recognize its limitations in terms of the issues which divide, as well as unite, women as a group (Patai, 1991; Judith Stacey, 1991). Jenny Douglas (1992) has recently raised these issues in relation to research on the health of black women, noting that: 'White feminist researchers . . . fail to address the issue of white women interviewing black women. There is an assumption that the shared experiences uniting women outweigh the differences in relation to race and class' (p.39).

Alongside this challenge to the white ethnocentrism of much research to date, we would also stress that it is important for feminist researchers to recognize differences in relation to age. In this context, we are aware of the implicit contradictions for ourselves, as women in midlife, writing a book which seeks to give a voice to the experience of older women. Thus, in general research terms, it is vital that ways are found both of articulating the varied dimensions of the individual lives of older women, and of linking them with wider social, economic and political contexts.

The lives of older women: strengths and challenges

Drawing the above strands together, it is possible for us to summarize what we see as the major gaps and strengths in these perspectives, and to identify some of the challenges which they pose for understanding the lives of older women.

The demographic changes we have discussed have led, in recent years, to a growing concern with the older population. Some commentators would have us believe that, as a group, older people represent an increasing burden on society. They are portrayed as economically unproductive, increasingly frail, and especially vulnerable in terms of mobility, capacity for self-care and their proficiency in carrying out domestic and other tasks (OPCS, 1987a). The fact that the majority of older people are fit and healthy and live independent lives out in the community has been obscured by a veritable avalanche of research focusing on the 'problems of old age'.

As we have seen, older women greatly outnumber their male counterparts. Thus, the extent to which we regard older people as a burden and a social problem is going to have disproportionate implications for the lives of older women. An alternative outlook, and one to which the contributors to this book subscribe, is that this is both an inappropriate and unnecessarily alarmist view. It highlights and reinforces the negative stereotyping which pervades the lives of older women, and devalues not only their past contributions but also their existing capabilities and potential.

In addition, British work carried out to date within life-course, gerontological or feminist perspectives suffers from a number of weaknesses. We would argue that, with some of the exceptions already referred to, they have each failed to fully address the experiences, structures and processes which mould and shape the lives of older women. Put simply, our contention is that the life-course perspective has been blind on two crucial counts; in terms of gender and in terms of age. Likewise, gerontological perspectives have been largely gender-blind; while feminist perspectives have in turn been age-blind. These 'blind spots' are all the more lamentable given the various strengths and common elements which these approaches share.

This book represents our modest contribution to the dialogue. It is our belief that the perspectives we have outlined above challenge us on many levels, and that they have the potential within them to help us articulate what it is really like to be an older woman in late twentieth century, multicultural Britain.

In no particular order, we now draw out half a dozen of the issues we regard as crucial to the thrust of this book. First, all these perspectives place varying degrees of emphasis on process, whether it be at an individual, group or societal level. Through an enhanced understanding of the processes which fashion the lives of older women, it should be possible to better counter the discrimination and marginalization many of them experience. Second, all these perspectives draw their inspiration from different disciplines and, in so doing, have the capacity to provide us with a richer, holistic and multidisciplinary picture of life for older women. This in turn should enable us to unravel some of the complexity and flexibility these women demonstrate, as well as highlight the interconnections between facets of their individual and collective lives. Third, these perspectives challenge us to look at the positive as well as the negative aspects of old age, and suggest that our pathological view of older people in general, and older women in particular, needs to be countered by a focus on 'normal' ageing and on the variety of lifestyles which exist in old age. Here, it will be important to examine topics such as leisure, education and sexuality alongside our more 'traditional' gerontological concerns with issues such as caring, the nature of dependency and retirement. Fourth, amassing a body of knowledge about the lives of older women has significant implications for both practice and policy over the course of the next few decades. For example, it challenges us to consider different ways in which professionals might have to work with older women, as well as the distinctive skills they will need: issues we take up in the concluding chapter. A fifth area concerns the enduring theories and models on which we still rely. As we have already noted, many of them are male orientated and ethnocentric in both conception and application. We now need urgently to analyse and criticize this received wisdom, applying, for example, feminist theory to our considerations of age. Finally, the perspectives we have outlined have important implications for the ways in which we might conduct research and investigations of different kinds. Whilst agreeing with Graham Fennell and his colleagues (1988) that there is no single correct way to undertake research, our immediate inclination would be for gender and ethnically sensitive biographical approaches. Large- and small-scale studies would, in our view, offer one way to help counteract the current invisibility of older women.

Despite this invisibility, older women continue to live out intricate, difficult and enriching lives, struggling hard to overcome sexist, racist and ageist attitudes. It is the emergence, recognition and acknowledgement of this diversity and heterogeneity that we hope to convey in the following chapters.

In Chapter Two, the reader is presented with an immediate example of the benefits of the life-course approach we endorse throughout the book. By means of five specially commissioned biographical interviews with older women, Joanna Bornat, the coordinator of this chapter, provides a sensitive insight into the life stories of women from differing social classes: women who are distinctive in their ethnic origins; who are widowed, divorced or never-married; and who have differing lifestyles. Together, these stories yield important insights into the relations between personal experiences and the wider historical backcloth against which these women have lived out their lives. With their permission and blessing, each of our chapters opens with a quotation taken from the transcripts: quotations which we believe provide a unifying thread to the themes and issues we discuss and which illustrate, in their own words, what women bring to their old age.

With Chapter Three, we move into a consideration of what might be regarded as the more 'objective' dimensions of ageing. Dulcie Groves discusses women's relation with the formal economy and the world of work. She details the origins and consequences of women's lifelong dependent economic status, showing how their employment patterns, the current pension system and social policy relating to retirement and social security, have all contributed to the impoverishment and inequality which older women experience.

These issues are considered again in a different context in Chapter Four, when Moyra Sidell examines the health of older women. The gender differences in mortality and longevity noted earlier have important health consequences for women. For example, they appear in old age to suffer from more chronic and disabling conditions than men, and to make greater use of formal health services. Differing explanations for these gender differences are explored and analysed, alongside a discussion of issues including menopause, osteoporosis and the use of drugs and medication. Positive elements of women's health and wellbeing are also considered, including the growth of preventive and self-health-care practices.

Ways of enhancing women's mental wellbeing in later life are also of concern to Dorothy Jerrome who, in Chapter Five, examines the importance of relationships, friendships and sexuality in the mainten-ance of a positive self-identity. In the context of dramatic changes to the structure and constitution of family life, she highlights the value older women place on social networks and the significance of female friendships. This is developed into a concluding consideration of the nature of intimate relationships which exist amongst women in old age.

In Chapter Six, Gillian Dalley takes up the theme of women's caring nature, examining both their caring roles and the development of community care policies. She critically reviews the now substantial body of writing on these issues, and lays particular emphasis on revealing the reality of care from the perspectives of both carers and the older women they care for. We know that throughout the life course women take greater responsibility for caring, and this has serious implications for their command of various resources.

One of the key resource issues is highlighted by Sheila Peace in Chapter Seven. Here, she explores the existing and potential range of accommodation options available to older women. From a life-course perspective she shows how housing careers are changing in response to differing economic, social and political pressures: pressures which up until now have dictated that women's prime realm is within the private world of the household. She examines what home and com-munity really mean for today's older women, and discusses the impor-tance of related dimensions such as access to transport, mobility and communication, in enabling them to live independent lives.

In Chapter Eight, Miriam Bernard and Kathy Meade address this notion of independent lifestyles by examining the leisure and edu-cational potential of later life. We show that despite the now popular image of retirement as a period of leisure and pleasure, very few older women currently engage in what might be regarded as traditional educational and leisure activities. The reasons for this are many and varied, and we discuss three key sets of life-course constraints which we believe prevent older women developing a Third Age lifestyle of their choice. In particular, we focus on the effects of gender divisions in the domestic sphere; the influence of age and generation in relation to issues such as access to education; and gender-based social and economic restrictions such as lack of transport, fears for personal safety and inadequate financial resources.

These discussions of the cumulative impact of gender- and age-based discrimination over the life course echo the arguments of earlier chapters and lead us, in Chapter Nine, to a consideration of how they might be tackled. Together with Anthea Tinker, we look at a framework for challenging older women's dependent status, for combatting income inequality and material poverty, and for pursuing an equitable sharing of resources. Our argument here is that we need to urgently rethink the values, purposes and direction of the policies which impinge on women's situations as a necessary prerequisite for any concrete and lasting change in the quality of their lives in old age.

Conclusion

An introductory chapter is, by necessity, selective. What we have attempted to do is outline the conceptual basis for the book, arguing that our existing theories and frameworks need to be critically reassessed, since they fail to fully address the experiences of women in general, and older women in particular. We have shown too that, demographically speaking, ageing is very much about older women but that, as yet, we have little information which enables us to differentiate amongst this population along key dimensions such as race and ethnicity. Using elements from life-course, gerontological and feminist perspectives, we contend that an integrated life-course approach is necessary to counteract the invisibility of older women and to convey both the dynamism and complexity of their lives. Only in this way will we begin to redress the problem-oriented notions we have of old age, and reveal the strengths and positive attributes of older women alongside their undoubted difficulties.

2   Life experience

Joanna Bornat

Introduction

This chapter brings together five life stories: accounts given by older
women. Any book written by younger women risks sounding
detached, lacking the voices, knowledge and experience which distinguish older women. The idea was that I should invite some older
women to talk about their lives, making a personal narrative to parallel the other chapters in this book. The accounts, which I taped in
five interviews, are individually unique, yet they fall in with many
patterns of women's lives. Joan, Pat, Charanjit, Ray and Olga talked
to me about their experience as girls and women, as members of
particular social classes, with experience of race and ethnicity, as
family members, and as workers, paid and unpaid. Their life stories
illustrate what women bring with them to their old age.

These women come from quite varied and distinctive backgrounds.
Only five, they are in no sense an objectively constructed or representative sample. Two of the five I had interviewed before, about aspects
of their lives. One I knew as a semipublic figure, the other two were
introduced to me by a daughter and a mutual friend. Between them
they represent a wide range of statuses: they are single, divorced and
widowed; they are English, Welsh, Italian and Asian; they are upper
class and working class. As they told their stories it became obvious
that there were many overlaps in their experience. Pat, for example,
I knew as a cycle-shop owner. Growing up in Wales, her first language
was not English. Charanjit I had first got to know as the main carer
of her sick husband, living in a council flat. When she began to talk
about her childhood I realized that she was the first person I had
ever heard pronounce the word 'phaeton'. She grew up in what is now
Pakistan, the daughter of a wealthy cotton ginning factory owner.

As an interviewer I always find myself much in awe as I listen to
older people's life experiences. They seem to have done so much,
met challenges, and of course sit there as skilful survivors. When it
came to representing hours of tape this sense of inequality still dominated me. I wanted this chapter to be the result of a collaboration
between five contributors and an editor. I have tried to present the

way each has talked about her life so that their needs as authors meet with the objectives of this book. Inevitably this has meant making hard decisions about what to choose from 400 pages of transcribed speech.

In my role as editor I wanted their voices, excerpted though they are, to be as free as possible from commentary and analysis. I decided on a way to link these lives which would be as unobtrusive as possible. The result is that there are no academic references in this chapter. I felt that footnotes to other sources would distance these voices, making them sound like subjects for analysis rather than authors. I also chose not to organize the excerpts in themes, such as childhood, health, housing. Instead, I have organized their words around issues which focus on the contribution which a life-history approach can make to an understanding of older women's lives. Looking through the interview transcripts I came up with four possible benefits.

First, an interview which focuses on personal experience turns the table on the investigator, the younger woman, and makes the older woman the expert in the process. She talks about something she has first hand knowledge of: her life and the awareness and observation she has accumulated. The stories told are part of the lives of women who have experienced the greater part of the twentieth century. What younger women know as history these women experienced as life. Their accounts bring to light alternative perspectives on war, peace, nationalism and the postwar consensus.

Second, these accounts draw on individual witness, highlighting, underscoring and validating statistics and generalizations which otherwise may feel impersonal and general.

A third benefit is the contribution which life histories make to the recognition of difference and the significance of the unique. Each account is a reminder of the heterogeneity present in later life. Awareness of the totality of life experience means reviewing and reframing understandings of the state of being older and of choices and decisions which women make.

The fourth aspect highlights the giving of a life-history as an emotional experience, sometimes unexpectedly so, with childhood anger, adult grief, passions, sorrows and happiness recalled. An opportunity to talk about a whole life also demonstrates the range of skills and knowledge which older women possessed, or still possess, but which they may have few opportunities to display as they grow older. Emotions humanize accounts of being older and, perhaps more important, they reveal something of the powerful inner lives of older women.

Before I look at the four contributions which a life-history approach can make I want to talk briefly about the interviews and introduce the five women who offer their life stories.

The interviews

This chapter is the combined production of six people; a writer and five speakers. It condenses the whole process from interview to write-up. An interview is not without limitations. There may be differences of age and class and, inevitably, there will be differences of experience which may affect an older woman's sense of power or control while she is talking. However friendly and informal, an interview cannot be the same as a conversation. It has a product, an account, which one person takes away, either on tape or as notes. It has a formal beginning and an end that means that it may leave things unsaid, ideas unspoken. It is usually a one-way process of questioning, with one person dictating the direction and pace.

Although these limitations are important, I feel that they are more than matched by the striking contribution which voices make to understanding and interpreting. Even in transcription, copied down from tapes, the emphases, inflections and emotions of the accounts from Pat, Joan, Charanjit, Ray and Olga inject cultural and social realities which can only enrich an awareness of the process of becoming an older woman.

This chapter is the end product of a paring down process, doing no justice to the lives portrayed in the interviews. To an extent it has been a shared process. Everyone knew the purpose of the interview, how it would be used eventually, and why it was important. Everyone had a chance to comment and amend what is included here. The interviews put me in the position of someone who is listening and learning. I want to move on by introducing each person briefly. I have tried to keep quotations from the interviews as long as possible so that Joan, Pat, Charanjit, Ray and Olga's words and meanings are more complete and their voices prevail.

Joan is 79 and was born in Somerset. She had an older brother and sister. Her father was a 'small landowner squire'. She was educated at home by governesses until the age of 14, when she was sent to boarding school. She remembers seeing her parents about once a day as a rule and says she never really got close to her mother until her own middle age. Despite what seems like a life of privilege, she says she suffered from loneliness in her early years:

'. . . I think we played tennis in the summer, but I was very bad at that. I didn't enjoy that much. I liked everything to do with nature, I used to you know, wander about the fields and woods, rather by myself, and sort of study things like that. I was a bit of a loner, because of the situation I suppose really. I didn't make friends really until I, I eventually did when I went to boarding school, but I found it difficult. I would have liked them.'

After boarding school Joan lived in London. During the war she nursed, married and had the first of her three children. A few years after the war she divorced and eventually moved to live in the house she still lives in which is in a small town in Hertfordshire. Her children are married and she now has grandchildren.

Pat is 76 and grew up an only child in Wales before moving to Somerset with her parents, who owned a smallholding and poultry farm. As soon as possible she left home to get a job in London. At 16 she worked as a cook–maid, and later became a waitress. Work was only a means to an end for Pat. Her one passion in life has always been bikes and cycling:

'There was nothing in my life, only cycling, for years and years and years. I didn't do anything else. We used to have a club dinner once a year, but I didn't dance you know. I couldn't dance. But I used to go a lot on my own. I used to go right up to Stoke-on-Trent and I used to go to the Lake District, get soaking wet, and come back in the middle of the night to Birmingham. There's a café in Birmingham, an old lady she was, she was lovely. Ma Benson we used to call her . . . it was two o'clock in the morning I knocked at her door. She used to have a gun under the pillow. She used to come to the door, she used to say, Who's there. You'd say, It's me Ma. And she said, Oh come in, come in. So in we went and she was ever such oh, she was in her seventies, late seventies, but she did cyclists for years and years.'

Pat worked for a cycling shop in North London and eventually owned her own business. She retired when she was 70. She has been married twice, once briefly in the Second World War, then divorced. Her second marriage, just before she retired, ended after only four and a half years when her husband died. She had one son who got married. She has not seen him for some time.

Charanjit is 74. She grew up in an area between Lahore and Karachi, which was then a part of colonial India. She grew up in the Sikh religion. Her father owned cotton ginning factories and she and her two brothers and sisters were at first educated at home. She was married at 18 to a young Sikh lawyer who later became a political journalist. In 1958 she followed her husband to England with their two children. They had various jobs in shops and factories, finally both finding employment in the civil service. Her husband became ill with Parkinson's disease in his late fifties. She nursed him until he died. She lives on her own in a council flat, but spends long weekends at her son's house an hour's journey away across London. She has grandchildren and great grandchildren. She looks back on the changes in her life in terms of her own shifting independence:

'*Because over here I used to say what I thought. Before that I never said anything. Whatever he said I obeyed. But when we came to this country, I think I became a little bit different. I don't know why. He used to say when he was sick, Oh you are different now. You don't love me as much as you used to do. I said, Yes of course I do. But now I think I can do things. Before I didn't think I could. But I was always in favour of doing something. Not cooking or anything like that. When I was in Sargodha, then I used to go as a volunteer, to teach in school. I wasn't taking any money, but I used to teach poorer people or things like that.*'

Ray is the youngest of the five, at 66. She was born on the outskirts of Halifax in West Yorkshire. There were four children in the family, although her younger brother died in an accident as a baby. Her early memories are of poverty. Her father worked mainly as a boiler firer, her mother took in washing. Ray has never married and now lives with her sister in a council flat. She has worked all her life. Looking back there was only one time when she felt well off:

'*After the war when, in the 1950's . . . we went on a holiday. First holiday we'd ever had. And we went on a boat on the River Severn in Avon. On a launch you know, a cabin cruiser. And that was nice. And then I suppose when we were working and then I used to go down to my friends in Bognor. But then you see, our parents were poorly, and there was only me working, well we started going backwards way. And then, to be quite candid, in the last ten years, since this government came in, it's just gone down and down.*'

Olga is 72 and grew up with her seven sisters and three brothers, a member of the Italian community of Clerkenwell, London. Her mother had been a court dressmaker and sometimes acted as interpreter in the local courts. Her father was a skilled marble floor layer and later in life ran a café. She met and married her husband during the Second World War while she was working as an oxyacetaline welder. Her first three children were born in the war years and just after. Her last daughter was born as she was reaching 50. Her husband died five years later. She lives in a council flat in Hackney, North London, and is in daily contact with at least one of her daughters. Olga's story is full of the detail of her family life, her parents' and her own. Being raised as Italian taught her some hard lessons which she still uses:

'. . . *on the bus, on the ambulance, when we're going to the clubs, we've got a black driver and we went to the Tea Dance last Friday, and we'd all been stuck indoors because of the snow, and we was eager to get out, none of us had been out for nine or ten days. And*

*of course the bus came to take us. And we went . . . to an elderly
woman that doesn't go out much. And the driver said to me, he said,
when she opened the door and found he was there, she didn't want to
come. He said I know how she feels . . . She was really frightened of
him and he knew it. And I felt sorry for him . . . everybody thinks
they're villains, everybody thinks they're dirty. And as I say to him,
Look I had all that when I was young. We weren't Italian, we were
dirty Italians because you were Italian you were dirty.'*

Life experience as history

These five life stories between them cover the major events of twentieth century history. At the same time they provide a parallel narrative which is one of twentieth century women's history. The life
stories document changes of which Olga, Ray, Joan, Pat and Charanjit have been a part. They can claim ownership in the public events
of official history by superimposing their own experiences and perspectives.

Charanjit has her own account of Partition in India. She had sym-
pathies for the nationalist movement for Indian independence and
these were strongly reinforced by her husband's outspoken beliefs
and actions. Partition, however, was not what they had expected or
desired. As Sikhs living in Lahore, later to become part of Pakistan,
they were directly affected. Her account details the personal disruption and disaster that political and religious divisions can cause.
Forced out of Lahore, they left their Muslim colleagues, neighbours
and workers and their printing press and travelled by army truck to
safety. Her memory is of a husband who was 'so brave, he was never
afraid, never afraid in his life' as he stood with a gun on the truck.

Eventually they reached Amritsar where to start with they lived
with their two young children in an office belonging to a friend. Later
her whole family managed to leave, but by then they had lost all
their possessions. A Muslim refugee family was living in their house
in Lahore and when her husband went back he was not even able to
collect their family photographs.

Olga's experience of war in Europe was to work in an environment
which had been previously all male. At home the family learned the
hard way what being classified as an alien meant. Her father had
refused to take out British nationality on a point of principle, even
though he had fought on the British side in the First World War:

*'They took my father's bicycle away, and things like that. But, and
when we went to the shelter of a night-time, when the air raids were
on, we would all go to the shelter, at first we sheltered in Kings Cross
Road, but we had so much abuse there because we were Italian that,*

my aunt lived nearer Holborn, and she said, Why don't you come and sleep in the Holborn tube, where most of the Italians were. So we used to go there. And my father wasn't allowed to come out, because he was an alien. He couldn't come out after nine o'clock at night. And he used to have our breakfasts all ready and in the winter a big fire made for us . . . And then, living in Grays Inn Road with a barber's shop was an Italian man, Mr Evangelista. And he was the head of all the fascists in this country, Italian fascists, which my father never involved himself for, because he was more of a left wing, you see. And Mr Evangelista used to parade past our shop, to annoy my father, with all the fascists behind him. Churchill decided that any Italians over 75 were no risk to the country. And what annoyed my father so much, the biggest fascist in this country was allowed to do exactly what he liked because he was over 75, and yet my father that had no fascist ideas at all was restricted from going out, we didn't have a wireless, we didn't have a bicycle, if we'd have had a car that would've been taken away from us. To our family, it seemed so ridiculous.'

As a woman of 49, in the peacetime 1970s. Ray had her own experience of employment chances. She fancied a change from office work in a mill and applied for a job at the Electricity Board as a meter reader:

'I thought, ooh, a complete change, I'll be out in the fresh air and all that . . . I said, I've come to apply for the job. So she sent for the manager. So he said, Well, you can fill your application form in now. So I did. Then he interviewed me. And he said, Very unusual a woman coming after this job. He said, It entails a lot of walking. I said, I'm in a hiking club, I said, I've walked up to fifteen miles, over moors, in a snowstorm. So he said . . . You've got to go out in all weathers. I said, I've got a raincoat and a pair of wellingtons, and trousers. So he said, It's a complete change. I said, I'm looking for that . . . And I mean, I was reasonably fit . . . So anyway he said, I must warn you . . . do you like dogs? I said, Yes, I'd be afraid of a vicious dog. But I said, I've always had a good relationship with dogs, I said . . . So he said, Well I must tell you that most of our meter readers leave because they've been chased or bitten by dogs . . . So he said, We'll let you know. So anyway they said they were sorry. But I am convinced it was because I was a woman. It had nothing else to do with it. I mean I could walk as good as anyone else . . . I could have done that, I felt sure I could.'

Reading through and listening to the accounts it seemed to me that each had their own perspective on what are regarded as public accounts of history. Charanjit saw the Partition of her country following independence in 1947. Her part was that of a wife, mother, Sikh and nationalist. Olga has personal experience of being on the margins of British wartime society. Ray experienced the reality of a labour market imposing inequality and immobility, literally in her case, on women. But their accounts are more than simply factual. The language they use, their choice of words and phrases, underline how they feel now and felt then about what they describe.

The individuals behind the statistics

In their detail, life stories provide access to aspects of daily life that are rarely documented, highly individual accounts that match what may be generally described and numbered. These may be inaccessible areas, difficult to speak about. In terms of a whole life they help to explain and illustrate why particular paths are chosen, what chances were open to each.

A feeling that they were innocent, compared with the younger women of today runs through some of the accounts, like Charanjit's: 'My childhood was innocent, when I had a period I didn't know what it was. I was 14 years old and I don't know what it was. I was crying.' That innocence, particularly innocence of the facts of life, may seem difficult for younger women to understand today, given descriptions of lack of space or large families. Olga talks about her parents' marriage and helps to explain how young people were kept ignorant or sheltered. She provides access to an understanding of private feelings:

'*They were wrapped in themselves but, er—and yet you say that, I never heard a word of endearment from either of them to each other. Alec was Alec and Mary was Mary. And that was it. I've never seen my father ever say Dear and on occasions when he went away to working laying floors, because he had to go all over the country laying floors, er, the cards would come, never had Dear Mary on it. Mary, never had Dear.*'

And they never kissed one another?

'*Never in front of us. Never. We never. And my mother, if she was having a wash in the living room, and my father walked in, he wasn't allowed in. He used to go and sit in the bedroom. No, he didn't see my mother undressed in front of us.*'

Explaining how families survived on low incomes becomes easier with first-hand accounts like that of Ray. In her case, 'family' meant her parents, the three surviving children and her father's father:

'. . . *he was born before his time, my granddad. He read a lot, and he got ten shillings pension and he collected that on Friday. And*

*sometimes when we went to school in the morning, it was twopence
halfpenny a week for milk, if you had milk, you know, well on
Friday morning we never have twopence halfpenny left. So we didn't
get any milk. And my mother used to be making fatty cakes in the
frying pan, didn't she, for our breakfast, on Friday morning, cause,
you know, the cupboard was bare. And then at dinner time when
we got home there was a great stew and my dumplings. And my
granddad had got his pension, you see. I used to wonder where it
all came from.'*

The interviews provide evidence which links directly to what is
revealed from more formal survey methods of research and questioning about older women's material resources and opportunities. At
one level this is an opportunity to validate statistical evidence. At
another level they provide frameworks for understanding how
decisions are reached within the limitations or opportunities dictated
by family, gender, race and class.

Only Pat lived quite independently of her family as a young worker
in the years running up to the Second World War; first as a cook,
later as a waitress. Joan too was living in London at this time but,
as she describes it, her parents 'did support me a bit as well'. She
drove up and down to Somerset at weekends and 'quite liked going
home'. To break away from family support, or control, involved
risk-taking and convention breaking for young women. Pat's mother
was not happy with her daughter's choice of lifestyle:

*'She wasn't like me. I was a tomboy, according to her, you know. My
cousin Valmay, which was my aunty's daughter, she liked her all right,
because she was kept home for years and years, just worked in the
shop . . .'*

Staying within the control of your family of origin or making your
own, through marriage, had distinct repercussions for the four others.
As a single woman, Ray became the breadwinner when times became
hard for the family in the 1950s:

*'. . . by this time Jessie (sister) had left, she'd gone to look after an
aunt who lived away, and she was there with her for about twenty
years, she had spondylosis and whatnot, of the spine. And my brother
had married. And so there was just my wage and my dad's wage in
summer, but nothing in winter . . .'*

Staying in the family, as a woman, meant that you had access to
family resources. For Joan these resources included a roof over her
head after the divorce which left her supporting three young children
without a profession or the means to buy a home:

'. . . *when my father died everything was left in a trust for my sister and brother and me to inherit eventually. And somebody suggested that the trust might invest in a house and let it to me, as an investment, as opposed to having it in the bank or something. And I wrote to the trustees and they came up with the idea. My mother agreed with it too. The idea was that the money was invested in bricks and mortar, and was rented to me.*'

Now she pays no rent, since her mother died the house is 'just part of the trust'. If your family has limited resources, then the move into retirement is likely to involve further material loss. As Ray explains:

'*We've nothing, apart from the pension, and my company pension. I did opt to take a lump sum in lieu. I could have had a bigger pension. But where we lived till our parents died . . . it was a council house, a big one . . . when we moved here (the flat) we had six pounds between us. That's all. So I retired about eighteen months later . . . with the money I got, we had to decorate, nothing would fit . . . (now) that money is gone . . .*'

Ray's and Joan's accounts illustrate the powerful effect of social class on the position of older women. Differences in their accommodation can be explained in class terms. Interestingly, neither is a wealth owner in her own right, a comment perhaps on the economic status of women.

Olga had to postpone her independence from family financial responsibilities until her youngest daughter, born when she was 48, just five years before her husband died, had graduated from university and got a job:

'. . . *that pension is all mine, . . . and you know what I mean, I've had to think to myself, Shall I buy a dress for myself? No, Sylvie needs something. But now it's all my own. It's all my own and, although it's only forty-nine pounds a week, it's mine. I've got to pay my poll tax, I've got to pay a little bit of rent, 'cos I'm on income support, but I can manage.*'

Pat feels that her life is quite different to that of her parents at her age:

'*Oh yes, they didn't have any more when they were older than when they started really. I mean, you know, very little money than when they started. But I mean, I've worked hard for my money, I've worked very hard. I mean, but I liked the work, it wasn't a job I didn't want. I mean, if somebody wanted a pair of wheels on a Saturday morning I would get them done if I was up till one doing them.*'

Working hard and moving up to London are, for her, the main reasons why she is experiencing, relative to her parents, an affluent old age. She escaped the restrictions of parents and family, exchanging them for what she feels was a career of her own choice and making.

Illustrating differences

Life-history accounts reveal the different experiences that women bring to later life. Although there are continuities with younger women, older women have lived through different times, which offers a contrast with their situations today. Earlier experiences may account for the ways in which major life changes such as caring and being cared for are dealt with. Quite coincidentally, Joan and Charanjit lived in experimental collective settings during or after the Second World War.

Charanjit describes her experience:

'. . . *they were doing new experiments in Preetnagar . . . what they were doing was that we should live together with each other, and there should be, well, different values. There was one kitchen. And we were all families, twenty families started this thing. And they took some, they took over the land, and they were doing different experiments. Our leader was Mr Gurbakhash Singh . . . we didn't do the cooking, servants did the cooking, but we were there to supervise things, and whenever—it was like a canteen you could say,—whenever we met each other, there were so many things (to discuss), people used to come and have lunch together, at night we got together. And there were so many, not political things, so many meetings, especially journalism and things like that . . . very happy days I remember.'*

Several thousand miles away just north of London, a few years later in 1946, Joan and her husband and two little daughters were also experimenting in living:

'. . . *we joined a community. I had Jo and Miranda her sister by then. And we lived with eight other families in a big country house . . . And they were all sort of left-wing and most of them were rather bright sort of serious people . . . We had a bedroom and a children's room and a bathroom for each family. And then we shared everything else. Looking after the house, and helped each other with the children, and the garden and things like that. It was a real proper community. We grew our own food and things to a certain extent. Most of the husbands were working in London. One or two of them were working at home . . . One was an MP, two were MPs actually. Socialist MPs. And two*

*were barristers and a film producer and a couple of publishers . . .
they were considerably brighter than me I think . . . I enjoyed it very
much while it lasted.'*

It was both Charanjit's and Joan's husbands who ended their involvement in the experiments. Charanjit's husband had differences with
Gurbakhash Singh over the sale of land at Preetnagar. Joan's husband developed an ulcer and was advised to take outdoor work, but:

*'There was a certain lack of . . . the average family unit. I think
the men missed that more, they wanted, you know, their wives
running around after them and the children doing what they were
told! But I think the children enjoyed it and the women certainly
did . . . I suppose part of their dream coming back from the War
was just that—having a cosy little home, because they'd been so
much with other people. More than the women had of course, on
the whole. But then they must have wanted to come in the first
place, or they wouldn't have come.'*

Despite their experience of communal living, neither has any desire
to change their living arrangements now. Joan explains her rejection
of what she has seen of communal living in old age:

*'It's going down, instead of—when I was in the other community, one
was on one's way up one thought. I don't want to, I'd sooner stay put
at the moment and keep going in any way I can.'*

Charanjit keeps her options open. She spends part of the week in
her own flat and part of the week at her son's house.
    Past experiences of caring and being cared for have left their mark
on each. For Pat there was no question of looking after her widowed
mother, they did not get on and her aunty lived near her. In contrast,
Ray and her sister Jessie could not imagine doing anything else:

*'. . . my mother looked after everybody, not just her own family. She
looked after loads of people, did my mother. And always there to help
people. She was kind. She was a kind person. And she never turned
anybody away, you know . . . And I thought, well, how can you send
somebody (into a home)? My mother wouldn't have wanted to go.'*

But Ray is clear that caring can 'kill the families off' and that 'let's
face it, it's the woman in the family, even if it's a married woman,
it's the woman who's doing most of it'. Charanjit would surely agree.
She cared for her husband, who was ill with Parkinson's disease, for
eight years until he died:

'. . . *it was very hard work. I would never say to anyone that they are not doing enough. Because you can't satisfy a patient. Whatever you do, the patient always thinks that it's not enough. Maybe I would be the same . . . sometimes I became a little bit upset when he wasn't happy . . . he was altogether a changed person. When he became sick he was not the same man as he used to be—always determined. When he became sick he was always very submissive and regretted the kind of man he had been . . . when he was suffering, he might say something to me, I noticed this because whenever he became upset he would say uncharacteristic things to me. Otherwise all through his life he never said anything bad to me . . . he suffered a lot but I did what I could for him.*'

The eight years Charanjit spent as the main carer of her husband have left her with fairly negative feelings about the ability of families to care:

'*Everybody has to go. Now it's always been my feeling that . . . I don't know what God will do with me . . . but my children will not do anything for me. I know. Because you see, nobody can do everything. You can't blame the children, it's because nobody can do everything through such a long illness. Because I suffered from doing this. And what I think is that it is very difficult to care for somebody for such a long time.*'

Ray and her sister Jessie are at the centre of a network of care and support: 'Well all of our lives we seem to have been looking after poorly people and it hasn't stopped now'. They list neighbours and relatives:

'. . . *Ronnie upstairs, he's been poorly a few times. Well, we have his key, we've to send for the doctor and that. And do his shopping and his washing. We always do his ironing. And then there's neighbours. There's a neighbour across, well, if we see his curtains aren't pulled back in the morning, we go across. Well, we ring him. He's a phone by his bed and if he's poorly we take him some tea over . . . I had two cousins up Pelham poorly, those neighbours were poorly. And somebody else was poorly and I was shopping for all the lot of them, through all that snow . . . And I mean you're forced to. You can't leave them.*'

Ray and Jessie are younger than Charanjit and although caring for their mother was exhausting—she was immobilized by a stroke and incontinent in her last years—they had each other for support. Charanjit did her caring alone, and while Ray and Jessie feel that they were returning and repaying kindness, her experience, as a wife, was that the illness changed her relationship with her husband, leaving her with unresolved feelings of sorrow and guilt:

'*Sometimes when he was suffering I thought, Oh it's all right, But it was very bad, I mean. And I'd think about sending him to a home, because I was thinking seriously about this . . . sometimes I said to him, I think I should send you because I can't pick you up. Because he fell down so many times. Then sometimes he didn't know his bed was wet, so I couldn't do anything. My energy wasn't enough for him. So I said two or three times, I want to send you to a home. I will come every day. Why don't you want to go? Then he became very sad . . . Now I think, yes, now that he's gone it was for my sake, because he felt very much that he was causing trouble.*'

Exposing feelings, revealing skills

Emotions humanize and flesh out accounts of growing older. Older women particularly suffer from a negative stereotyping which portrays their lives as emotionally narrow or deprived, or disconnected from the experiences of younger people. In the telling, feelings come through and the whole person emerges.

Pat's commitment to cycling originated in what she describes as a desperate need to get away from the countryside:

'*I'd lived in Somerset and I used to go out the fields and cry. I was so lonely down there it was terrible. I used to go out the woods and see all the animals in the woods and all that, on walks, on my own. But it was, if you've got no one to talk to when you finish school and all that, it's dreadful living in a place. Because I used to go out, clean the eggs and, you know, water the chickens, and we had quite a big chicken farm there, and ducks there, and geese there, and all that, nanny goats there. It was a proper country sort of thing. But it wasn't my thing.*'

She went with an aunt to London and found a job in service,

'*. . . then I got this job in Lyons . . . I was there ten years. And that was freedom, you know, you didn't have to go in at night, and you could go out on the bike on Sunday. I mean, I've been out at three o'clock in the morning and then come back for one with a ten-hour in Lyons. I've gone in there all sweaty, covered in sweat, and they say, Where you been? I say, Oh I've been down the Bath Road marshalling. I used to go down and marshall for the hundreds down there. The boys used to come round throw little pebbles at the window to wake me up if I wasn't up. You know, tiny pebbles . . . my friend used to say, What's that? I said, That's the boys outside. Ssh! Don't say anything. That's the boys out there, waiting for me. So I used to creep downstairs with my bike. She wasn't a cyclist, this girl, she was*' *just an ordinary person, you know. She used to go to Sunday School and all that.'*

Feelings about love and friendship are part of these accounts. Olga's parents are still important figures in her life as she tells it:

'*I am not ashamed that I had Italian parents, I had lovely parents, the best parents. And I was bragging once . . . I was bragging about the lovely parents I had, and afterwards a woman came over to me and she said, Not all of us had a good home life. And I realized I had been bragging. And I realized that people didn't all have that lovely home life.'*

The effects of women's lower pay, confinement to less-skilled jobs and restricted opportunities for advancement are well documented in statistics: these show the results to be relative financial inequality for older women compared with older men. What the statistics cannot show is how women feel about their experience of inequality. Ray is clearly angry:

'*When I retired, and I'd worked there twenty-seven years, I got nothing, nothing. And I didn't expect anything. But I'd worked hard, and in certain cases I'd saved the company money. And I'd once actually saved it from grinding to a halt . . . So I reckoned I'd earned my keep there. And from my workmates and my colleagues, yes, they collected, and they asked me what I wanted, and I said a duvet and covers and things. And they also brought flower arrangements and my friend at work, she bought me the book The Country Diary of an Edwardian Lady . . . So my workmates, yes I really was, I liked all the people I worked with . . . But I did work, for what, I'll tell you what. When I retired seven years ago my take-home pay was fifty-four pounds a week . . . at the time they used to be saying on the television that the average wage is a hundred and twenty pounds . . .'*

The exploration of a life history reveals differences in experience, and with these differences comes a wide variety of skills. Talking to the five, it became clear that between them they could assemble a powerful array of knowledge and abilities. Apart from their skills as carers, mothers, wives, activists and workers, they have specific knowledge from earlier phases in their lives. Charanjit worked as a teacher and was a radio announcer writing her own copy for a new radio station in the Punjab during 1948. Ray worked with an early computer in her anti-aircraft unit in Croydon, predicting the trajectory of enemy missiles. Later she worked in a carpet factory doing budget controls, graphs and 'things about production and targets'.

Olga ran a canteen at a college of further education and worked ˙
as a welder. Joan worked as a nurse during the war and later was
deeply involved in the early days of CND, taking part in marches
and sit-ins: 'I think I wanted to be involved in something that wasn't
just me, as it were. Causes, I think I found I wanted to be involved
in something that was going to be some good to somebody'. Pat's
knowledge of bikes was already legendary when she was a younger
woman:

'My governor gave me a wonderful reference. 'Cos I mean sometimes
the bloke would come in and he'd talk, Have you got this? An old
cog, would be years old. And I used to explain to him that he couldn't
use that on something or other, because this or that, and he used to
turn round and he'd walk away. One bloke walked away one day,
went up to the governor. And he said, Look, he said, what she don't
know about bikes, nobody knows. He said, She's told you what's
right, now get out. He wouldn't talk to him, because he tried to make
out I was a woman and I didn't know what I was talking about, and
all that. And what I was talking about was right. Because I mean, I'd
been in it since I was sixteen.'

Making connections

During Olga, Charanjit, Pat, Ray and Joan's lives there have been
significant changes for women in general. The growth of feminism in
social and political movements has altered perceptions about
women's status at home and at work. What do they have to say about
their lives now that they look back through changing times? What
do they have to say about women in society today?

Olga reflects on the differences between her own and her daughters' marriages:

'Oh I've made my own life and as much as my mother kept us under,
so did my husband keep me under. My children will never be under
their husband's thumbs like I was . . . the other day they were giggling
here. And I said what are you giggling at? And they said, We want to
know why you had such butch women. So I said, What do you mean?
So well Sylvia's . . . a trainee manageress where she is. And they call
her the Godmother. And . . . they call Jean Queen Jean, Queen . . .
We've waited on our men all our lives, us, my family you know. And
these girls don't . . . Jean got O levels for cookery but never cooks a
thing. John does all the cooking. She says, I work, I say, you letting
John do the cooking, but I work mum. You see?'

Charanjit worries about balancing women's independence with a need for children to be obedient. For her, women still have a central role within the family:

'I've always liked women to be independent. Not always sitting at home and just bringing up the children. I agree that bringing up children is a very very good job because you have to tell your children what's · wrong and what is—if a woman is always out and there's nobody to care for children, then the children don't care for you. But what's going on today is that children are becoming very careless. They don't agree with their parents, whatever they want to do they just do it.'

Pat's life has been unconventional in the sense that she stuck with one community, the cycling community and its ways, all her life. She lived in her cycling shorts in the early years, even though people could be narrow-minded. But it didn't bother her:

'No, because I didn't mix with anybody else, only cyclists. You know, they were all—all my friends were cyclists. And we'd all have shorts on, and we'd knock at their houses and pick them up . . . The neighbours would all take the curtains open and have a look. But we didn't worry about it, because it didn't worry us at all. We didn't interfere with them and Oh yes, you were frowned upon, with a lot of people in those—But then there were cafés the cyclists went into, and they got quite used to you. But you couldn't go into a pub like that at all. We only went into cycling cafés that we knew.'

In 1957 Pat opened her own shop. She started with £800, her savings plus £200 left her by her mother. 'The boys' did the shop out for her, built cupboards and whitewashed it. The fact that she was a woman starting in business on her own does not seem to have concerned her, what made the difference was the wheels, 'Well, if you hadn't been doing wheels, it wouldn't be bringing enough money in'. She has lived in the cycling community, becoming a celebrated craftworker in her own right, and spent most of her life as a single person. Perhaps this has been a form of protection for Pat, supporting her and insulating her from the persisting sharp edges of discrimination in the workplace and enabling her to avoid any limitation imposed by a marriage partnership.

Ray stayed single, but for her there was no protection from the inequalities of the labour market. Looking back now she is clear about the unfairness of it all:

'. . . when I think of the years I worked, and they had, when we were working, at the height of our working days, they had what they called a man's wage and a woman's wage. You were doing the same work. And getting a lot less for it. And it was accepted. People thought it

was only right. Because you're a woman you should get a woman's wage. I mean, people, married or single, married women, they should still get the equivalent wage. I don't care what the husband gets. I think it's a good thing. I mean, the modern woman today, I mean, I support all these things that they're trying to get today, because the women, in our day, they really were back numbers. After the War, of course, it was a lot better, and then, according to your circumstances, which you can't always alter. But women today, it's much better for women.'

She ties up some of the points in her life by involving herself in local and national activities. She joined Ex-Services CND before she retired. She has been arrested for cutting the wire at an airbase and explains her commitment in terms of her wartime experience, 'We knew people, soldiers and friends who were killed in the war. When you look in the local roll of honour and you see boys you went to school with in the roll of honour, you realize what the war's about.' Finally, Joan dates what she describes as 'a kind of feminism' in her own thinking from the time she lived communally with a group of left-wing people of about her own age. She has only really found it possible to follow her ideals in more recent years, although having these ideals helped her through the difficult times of her divorce and the struggle to bring up three children on her own. Since her late fifties, she has done a great deal of travelling round the world, and she is actively involved in causes that are important to her; the National Council of Women, Amnesty and Oxfam. Talking about older women she knows she says:

'I think most of my friends have vaguely the same ideas as I do. I think really the ones that have managed to go on being needed are much happier. I mean they've either done things, or their families need them, or somebody needs them. Once they get to the stage of not being needed and only wanting things for themselves, they get miserable. I've noticed that in some of my friends I suppose.'

Making connections means looking across lives, at phases through which we are all presumed to pass. For women, biology and married status seem to dominate the sequence of life phases, as girlhood is succeeded by courtship, marriage, motherhood, 'the change' and being a grandmother. But not all our five passed through all these stages at the same point in their lives. Olga became a mother at a time when Charanjit became a grandmother. Pat married again as others were encountering widowhood. Ray never married and Pat only briefly, on two occasions.

Nor has biology always determined how a life course has developed. Loneliness, which is so often associated with being single in later life, was something which both Pat and Joan experienced when they were young girls. Now older and both single, they are more in control of their lives and describe busy, fulfilled days. Although friendship networks may be determined by opportunities of work and marriage, outside political events have also shaped life courses. During the war years both Joan and Ray made friends who are still important to them, connections with earlier stages in their lives. These five lives, although shaped by similar life events, make their own particular connections.

Silences

I have highlighted four areas where I feel these life-history approaches illuminate our understanding of the lives of older women. Inevitably there are gaps in these accounts; stories that remained untold, reflections that did not surface during the interviews. A silence can be a sign of refusal, an unwillingness to divulge. It may suggest that during the interview we were close, but not intimately so. After all, although we are all women I was still aware that there were differences that we all displayed quite strongly: differences of class, knowledge, advantage, region, background, race, and of course age. And there was the question of context and timing. Talking to someone for the first time, a newcomer, in your front room, on a weekday morning, is not always a guarantee that you will feel like 'telling all'. I sensed all these barriers of context and difference and I found myself aware and respectful of them. I wanted the interviews to be self-motivated rather than prompted or drawn out.

One of the most obvious areas of silence was in accounts of health and wellbeing. None of the five offered me descriptions of their health. Only Ray mentioned poor health in connection with low points in her early middle years. Perhaps, contrary to popular stereotypes, health is not a constant preoccupation of older women. Leisure or time for oneself was also not an obvious focus which any of the five describe. Ray talks about walking and reading and Pat her cycling during the working years. Now that they are all retired they fill their days with many activities, some which might be described as leisure, like reading or watching videos. Others fit more properly into the context of learning and work, activities like education classes, meetings and caring.

For Charanjit, Olga, Pat, Ray and Joan, time out of paid work meant time to be with others who mattered, friends, causes, children, grandchildren, 'the boys'. Other people were the focus for leisure choices which the five made throughout their lives and to some extent still make today. If there is a silence around leisure, it is more to do with what women mean when they talk about time to do what they want to do.

Conclusion

Life-history accounts help to reveal what women bring to their old age: their experience; knowledge; passions; and decisions. They help the whole person to emerge from statistics or the distancing of differing generations and perspectives. Most important perhaps, I feel that they help us all to make connections and to distinguish what is unique and new from what is shared and continuous in our lives as women. What was it like this experience of talking about your own life? When we began to talk, Joan said she had never connected up her life into one account before. At the end she seemed to be saying that the experience had changed her: 'Done me a power of good I can tell you'.

3 Work, poverty and older women

Dulcie Groves

'. . . that pension is all mine . . . I've had to think to myself, Shall I buy a dress for myself? No, Sylvie needs something. But now it's all my own and, although it's only forty-nine pounds a week, it's mine . . . Jean, my other daughter, she pays the poll tax for me . . . And of course I've got no—my husband's firm, all the men wanted to go in for a pension, but the firm wouldn't agree to it . . . and I've never got any pension from anywhere I've worked . . . I've always had part-time jobs. So I never paid for a bigger pension. Sorry now, but I manage. I get by. I say to myself there's nothing I want in a hurry . . .'

(Olga)

Introduction

Women over 50 tend to be largely invisible in discourse about the financial circumstances of older 'people' despite the fact that older women are at far greater risk to poverty than older men. Such invisi-. bility helps to marginalize older women, some of whom are very poor indeed, especially if they have lived well on into 'old' old age. Older women will remain substantially at risk to poverty unless certain features of women's particular vulnerability to poverty in later life are exposed, analysed and, as far as possible, remedied. Part of that remedy lies in the greater economic empowerment of women.

Women's greater risk to poverty (however defined) in old age is directly related to the differential opportunities that women and men have to carry out paid work, to defer earnings for use in old age and to exercise choices about making financial provision for later life. A crucial determinant of available income and capital resources in later life is marital status, since retirement and widowhood benefits can be inherited through marriage: such benefits are lost on divorce. An individual's economic status is also influenced by the extent to which income and assets have been shared fairly in marriage and in the family of origin. Lifetime earnings and marital status also determine the extent to which people have the opportunities (or not) to make long-term savings or investments, including the purchase of owner-occupied housing as a capital asset which can be realized. Finally, some people inherit money, property or other assets, typically from parents or relatives. However, for most of us, it is our 'employment career' and that of our spouse/partner (if any) that are crucial in determining how adequate our income and capital resources prove to be in later life; the sheer length of old age, our own 'life course' and individual personal circumstances, together with external economic forces (such as the rate of inflation or economic recession), are also influential. In the past, women's opportunities have been far more restricted compared with men's: many inequalities and double standards remain.

This chapter begins by considering what is meant by the term poverty. It then focuses on trends in women's employment from the early twentieth century, the point at which some of the oldest women in the UK population became economically active. An exploration of the relation between women's paid work and their unpaid work in the home is then followed by a discussion of pension schemes and poverty among retired women. Last, attention is given to the employment status and experiences of the current generation of late middle-aged women, many still economically active but within sight of reaching 'pensionable age' at 60.

Conceptualizing poverty

Unfortunately it is very difficult to gain an adequate perspective of the extent of poverty among women. The problems inherent in trying to define poverty are many, and this situation is compounded when attempting to define poverty in relation to women. Peter Townsend (1987) has long argued for a definition of poverty which moves well beyond the concept of a 'poverty line' (a particular income level) to cover a far wider notion of 'deprivation': 'a state of observable and demonstrable disadvantage relative to the local community or the wider society or nation to which an individual, family or group belongs' (p.125). As illustrated in his major study of poverty, depri-vation extends beyond sheer 'income poverty' to encompass such variables as housing and environment, employment (or lack of it) and the paid workplace, as well as membership of groups commonly subject to forms of discrimination (Townsend, 1979). David Piachaud (1987) has elaborated further on the problems of poverty definition and measurement, encompassing social definitions of poverty (what the public defines as poor), the budget standard approach (the definition and costing of needs by experts) and the behavioural approach (defining the point at which poverty leaves part of the population demonstrably below the general standard of living).

The above material comes from a special issue of the Journal of Social Policy (1987) containing a number of articles on the definition of poverty which were subsequently criticized by Jane Millar and Caroline Glendinning (1989) for their failure to address gender issues. They argue that a whole new framework is needed for the analysis of gender and poverty, and proceed to document the economic disadvantages suffered by women compared with men and the structural causes of female poverty. Most importantly they contend that women are rendered invisible because statistical data is obtained from 'households' and 'families', making it impossible to disaggregate information on married women (Glendinning and Millar; 1987; 1991; Millar and Glendinning, 1989). Thus, while there is information available about women's earnings, much less is known about the extent to which household income is shared and allocated. Detail on lone women tends to be lacking in surveys because statistics on single, divorced and widowed women are, typically, conflated. There is a real need for research which addresses the causes of women's income poverty in old age as well as the wider causes of deprivation. Much more attention needs to be given to demographic variables of which parental status (with its crucial relation to economic activity for women) is a key example. Glendinning and Millar (1991) put the case for a far wider definition of poverty, encompassing not only income, but also access to goods, services and social activities, incorporating a costing of women's time.

Women's paid and unpaid employment in the twentieth century

Early in this century most women who worked in the formal economy had never married, although there were local areas where married women did typically do paid work (Elizabeth Roberts, 1988). Many women were required to leave their jobs upon marriage. Better paid occupations typically operated formal marriage bars, which affected women who were well qualified by the standards of the day, such as school teachers or civil servants. Many other employers had such bars or operated written rules (Jane Lewis, 1984; Meta Zimmeck, 1986). During the First World War many more women entered the paid labour market and held down responsible jobs, but most were not retained in the postwar period when marriage bars were even more rigorously applied and increasing numbers of single women wanted and/or needed paid employment (Gillian Braybon and Penny Summerfield, 1987; Lewis, 1984). What employers wanted was a continuous and eminently replaceable supply of young, cheap, female labour. For women who were really interested in their jobs, or could not afford to give them up, it was 'career or marriage'. Widows were sometimes employed, but divorcees had a very equivocal position, there being comparatively few of them and fewer still who publicly acknowledged their generally stigmatized status.

Audrey Hunt (1988) notes that married women often worked in 'ill-paid, arduous and filthy jobs, often as home-workers', early in the twentieth century, although 'To have a working wife constituted a social stigma for many a husband' (p.5). Some working-class wives, usually from necessity, earned money in the informal economy as 'daily' domestic workers. Indeed, between the wars domestic service was the occupation of last resort for large numbers of working-class women (Deirdre Beddoe, 1989). Hard-up middle-class wives might take in lodgers (of suitable status), do high-class dressmaking at home or give music lessons to children. Many of these jobs do not show up in census data (Roberts, 1988). It was most unusual for upper-class women to work at all, regardless of marital status: it can be argued that they were, in formal terms, the most ill-educated of women (Gillian Avery, 1991).

Single women were, typically, 'kept' by their fathers or other male relations in more affluent families, and one thread of women's emancipation can be traced in the rebellion of single women against enforced financial dependence on others. It was not only married women who were targeted for full-time domestic work: single women were expected to keep house for elderly parents or unmarried brothers (Lewis, 1984). Young women of all social classes were expected to live at home and their low pay was (erroneously) dictated by the expectation that all of them lived at home with their families and never gave financial support to other people. Between the wars it became more usual for single middle-class women to do paid work, especially when younger. And there were always some women who were an exception to these general rules, even concealing their true marital status to avoid the 'marriage bar'.

The rise of part-time employment

The Second World War brought many more married and some single women into the paid labour force and generally expanded employment opportunities for women. It also established part-time work for women (Summerfield, 1984), leading to the appearance of the part-time 'married woman returner' in the postwar period. After the war, a time of full employment, it became usual for women to stay in full-time employment immediately after marriage as there was a demand for female labour and marriage bars had been abolished in formal terms. Paid work became a near universal experience for young, single women. By the 1960s a pattern had been established whereby women, as a general rule, left paid work before the birth of their first child, after which time they remained at home until their youngest child was in full-time schooling. At this point part-time work became a popular option, favoured by employers: some women, however, preferred or were under pressure to delay their 'return' until their youngest child was in secondary school. Increasing numbers of part-time jobs were created which typically offered convenient hours but low pay and minimal occupational benefits, if any (Veronica Beechey and Tessa Perkins, 1987). A decade later in the 1970s all classes of women were 'returning', mainly to part-time jobs in the first instance, with some moving on to full-time work. However, even by the 1980s it was unusual for mothers not to take a few years out of the labour market while their children were young (some returning between births), while a minority of older married and single women left or remained outside the labour force or reduced their paid work commitments so as to care for incapacitated and/or elderly family members (Jean Martin and Ceridwen Roberts, 1984).

The employment experience of black women

The shortage of labour in Britain after the war was a major factor in the waves of migration from both the West Indies and the Indian subcontinent. Some women came by choice as young women and have grown old here, some came to join partners and, unable to return home, established families here, while others came in later life to join families already settled (Fenton, 1987). By and large, and certainly for the first generation, the patterns of women's paid and unpaid employment of their original homelands were continued here. West Indian women, like many working-class, white women, have held a high level of responsibility for the economic support of their households. Slavery and colonialism forced many West Indian men to seek work away from the family home, requiring women to make a living as well as run the home and rear children. In Britain in the context of low-paid jobs, the majority of West Indian women have maintained these roles, albeit without the support of the extended family network to help with child care (Jocelyn Barrow, 1982; Bryan *et al.*, 1985). Asian women migrants, many from rural backgrounds in the Punjab, also brought with them a history of contribution to the income-generating agricultural work on the household farm. This was set however within a rigid sexual division of labour under the authority of the eldest male. When this first generation of Asian women came to join their husbands in an urban environment, going outside the household to work, in for example factories or hospitals, was culturally less acceptable (Saifullah Khan, 1979; Wilson, 1978). The added need to learn English compounded this, and it appears that most women did not enter the labour market. There has been little research into their experience, but small-scale studies of older people from minority ethnic groups in Derby and Leicester indicated that nine out of ten women of South Asian origin had never been in paid employment (Bhalla and Blakemore, 1981; Mays and Donaldson, 1981).

Racial discrimination in the labour market exacerbated the sexual discrimination experienced by all women. Legislation passed to combat such discrimination included the Sex Discrimination Act (1975), the Equal Pay Act (Amended) 1984, and the Race Relations Act of 1976. Despite this, white people, and white men in particular, are consistently found in higher status jobs with higher earnings than women (Fenton, 1991). The 1985 Labour Force Survey also showed that since the 1970s unemployment among black women had risen faster even than that among white women, largely because they had been in unskilled jobs which are the first to be shed.

Common but unique employment histories

Thus, as can clearly be seen, each 'older woman' in the UK population has her own individual history of paid work, but is also a product of her times. If that 'older woman' is from an minority ethnic group or has physical or mental disabilities, she is likely to have experienced discrimination in the labour market over and above that experienced by women as a class. There are some very elderly women who have never done a paid job and were educated entirely at home. By contrast there are some women just turning 50 who have always been economically active as adults, returning to full-time work immediately after the birth of their children. The general rule is that the younger the woman, the more paid work she is likely to have done and the better qualified in formal terms she is likely to be. With the ending of the marriage bar, well-qualified women have tended to have higher economic activity rates across the age groups. However, the majority of women have experienced discontinuous employment over their lifetime employment careers (Hunt, 1988; Martin and Roberts, 1984; Heather Joshi, 1990).

Unpaid work and domestic roles

Women's relation with paid work has to be understood in the context of the unpaid work of the home. Despite the greater incorporation of women into the formal labour market since the Second World

War, at no time was it expected that the traditional gendered division of labour should be seriously disturbed. Men would continue to be defined mainly as the breadwinners and women as mainly responsible for the unpaid domestic work of the home (Sharon Witherspoon, 1988). Wives' earnings were typically defined as 'pin money', despite being spent mainly on necessities (Hunt, 1968). West Indian women; for example, used their wages to support family members here as well as in their country of origin. Moral strictures were directed at 'working mothers'. As Joshi (1989) has observed, 'economic autonomy is still a long way off for most British women' (p.157). Women work in a restricted number of job categories and their typically low level of earnings, especially if married, and their restricted hours of availability for work are, Joshi argues, 'in turn explained by two interacting factors, either of which is a sufficient condition for women's earnings to lag behind those of men: on the one hand the gendered division of labour, and, on the other, the unequal treatment of men and women in the labour market' (p.163).

With major inflation in the 1970s, and an increasing drive towards owner occupation in the 1980s, many married women's financial contributions to the household have become an ever more necessary and integral part of the family budget. Giving up paid work, for whatever reason, has become increasingly problematic for women, regardless of marital status. Married women cannot guarantee that their relationships will last. For women running households on their own and in some cases caring single-handedly for children or dependent adults, the loss of earned income can be catastrophic, with reverberations into later life and old age. Joshi (1987) has calculated that in 1980 'cash penalties of motherhood' were £135 000 in lost earnings: the knock-on effect for reduced pension entitlements are also considerable (p.127). Be that as it may, 'most women still subordinate their employment potential to the demands on their unpaid time and energy' (Joshi, 1990, p.125).

The resulting outcome of women's typical domestic and employment 'careers' is that up until the present time only a minority of women (married or not) can be said to be economically self-supporting in late middle age. Just as significantly, only a minority will have made, or been able to make, sufficient financial provision for an adequate pension or income *in their own right* in retirement. Pensions are built up over a 'working lifetime' of *paid* employment. Women in general have not been in a position to defer income for old age through the pensions systems, nor, for married women, has this been viewed as their responsibility. The next section outlines how this relation between women's paid and unpaid work has been reflected in the development of UK retirement and widows' pensions.

Women's access to retirement and widows' pension benefits

The history of UK pension provision in the twentieth century shows that both state and employers have not hesitated to compel male employees to contribute towards retirement and widows' pensions. However, the attitudes of pension providers towards women, and especially married women, have been equivocal to say the least. It is still the case that legally 'the husband's duty to maintain his wife is a normal incidence of marriage, whilst her obligation to maintain him results from abnormal and pathological situations' (Jan Pahl, 1989, p.24). Most older women of the present generation were brought up in the expectation that they would in due course marry and 'be provided for' rather than themselves be financially self-supporting, making provision for their own old age.

This present generation of older women has thus been the subject of public policies which placed responsibility for meeting the financial contingencies of old age (or widowhood) squarely in the hands of husbands. Such public policies have themselves been reinforced by domestic ideologies based on a traditional household division of labour, while public policies in their turn have influenced how men and women organize their domestic affairs and economic activity. Both state and occupational pension provision was designed with the needs of a 'male breadwinner' (and his dependants) in mind and has been adapted only slowly to meet the needs of women.

Poverty among elderly people (and especially women) was identified as a serious social problem in the late nineteenth century and means-tested old age pensions date from 1908. The first contributory old-age and widows' pension scheme (1925) was targeted at men and women with (in a context of unequal pay) average earnings or below and no employer's pension. This state pension was paid at 65 to men and women alike, regardless of whether they had actually retired: a pension was available at any age to widows of insured men (Dulcie Groves, 1983).

Before the First World War it was unusual for employed women, other than teachers or civil servants, to have access to an occupational pension scheme. During the interwar period, more private-sector employers offered pensions, but mainly as a fringe benefit available to salaried men. However, with increasing numbers of mature single women in the labour force following a huge male death rate in the First World War (coupled with an existing population imbalance), some private-sector employers did extend pension membership to women. Sometimes special (and inferior) women's schemes were offered. It was common for women to be admitted to membership of a 'unisex' scheme at a later age than men. Nor were the benefits offered necessarily equal to the men's, quite apart from the fact that women typically earned very much less than men during this period. When a census of employers' schemes was undertaken for the first time in 1938 there were five times as many men as women in membership (Groves, 1983).

Postwar developments

Following the Beveridge Report (1942), all members of the 1925 scheme were transferred into a new National Insurance scheme with entitlement to full pension provided that they continued to work for ten years (Ellis, 1989). This scheme incorporated a state retirement pension plus other benefits. Women paid a lower flat rate contribution than men, on the grounds that men (in general) earned more than women and male contributions (only) paid for dependants' benefits. A single person's full retirement pension was paid at a 'unisex' rate equal to a widow's pension. A married man's pension was payable at the same rate but also incorporated a married woman's (dependant's) pension.

Married women were given an inferior status within this new scheme, based on the explicit assumptions of the Beveridge Report that married women would be engaged mainly in the unpaid work of the home. Indeed, a husband's contribution automatically brought a dependent wife's retirement pension at 60 per cent of a full pension. Effectively, a married woman's full contribution bought only 40 per cent of a pension since it was not permitted for her to draw her own pension along with a dependent wife's pension. If a wife did paid work and paid full contributions so as to qualify for a pension in her own right at 60 (which she could defer until 65 if allowed to remain in her job), she had to be in insured paid employment for at least half of her married life, otherwise she lost *all* claim to entitlement, regardless of the number of contributions paid. All contributions made before marriage were lost if she failed this 'half test'. A further disincentive to paying full contributions was that married women only qualified for reduced unemployment and sickness benefits, on the grounds that they were housed and maintained by their husbands. Given such restrictive and complicated rules of entitlement, it is not surprising that the vast majority of employed married women exercised their right to opt out of paying full contributions. Most younger wives expected to leave paid work for an unspecified number of years upon motherhood. Yet there were cases in which it might well have been worth a wife continuing to pay, especially if she did in fact maintain a substantial record of paid employment and was older than her husband (Groves, 1983).

A married woman could not draw her dependant's pension until her husband reached 65 (or later) and drew his own pension. Pension levels were related to the number of contributions paid over a working lifetime and were abated (or not paid) in the case of an insufficient contribution record. The new means-tested National Assistance scheme acted as a safety net for people with insufficient National Insurance contributions, although wives could not claim in their own right.

After the Second World War employers were hungry for labour and extended occupational pension provision to the point where, by the end of the 1960s, most permanent 'good' non-manual jobs for men and many categories of male manual work (especially in unionized workplaces) carried occupational pension rights. More employers were offering widows' benefits. However, opportunities for women to belong to employers' pension schemes were more patchy. Full-time female public-sector workers had virtually no problems gaining access to their employer's pension scheme: normally this was required as a condition of service. But in the private sector it was still common until the mid 1970s for full-time women to be excluded from scheme membership or subjected to entry qualifications not imposed on men.

Many women found that their particular category of employment, in a gender-segregated labour market, simply did not carry entitlement to an occupational scheme. Employers noted that most married women opted out of the National Insurance scheme and consequently regarded women in general as uninterested in paying towards a retirement pension. With near-universal postwar marriage rates, it was assumed that most women would be 'provided for' in due course. Furthermore, it suited employers to exclude the growing number of part-timers (an overwhelmingly female category): their lack of access to fringe benefits made them attractive as cheap labour (Groves, 1987).

Recent changes

In 1975 major legislation was passed that at last began to redress the substantial discrimination against women in pension provision. The 1948 basic state retirement pension scheme was still in place, although in 1961 a second-tier earnings-related state pension scheme was introduced which gave poor benefits, especially for women. This unsatisfactory graduated scheme was replaced via the Social Security Pensions Act 1975 by another second-tier State Earnings-Related Pensions Scheme (SERPS). From 1977 all new female entrants to paid work and any woman who had left the labour market for more than two years had to pay full National Insurance contributions regardless of marital status. For the first time a system of credits towards the basic state retirement pension were awarded to men or women absent from the labour force (or earning so little as to be excluded from paying employee contributions to National Insurance) because they were caring for children (and in receipt of child benefit) or caring for severely incapacitated dependants (themselves in receipt of attendance allowance). Divorced women were allowed credits from their former husbands' pre-divorce National Insurance records. All this made it much more likely that, in future, women would at least qualify for a full state retirement pension at 60.

From 1978 employees were automatically included in SERPS (on top of the basic scheme) unless their employer opted to contract their particular class of employee out of SERPS and into an occupational pension scheme, which was required to incorporate widows' pensions. SERPS had an advantage for women (or men) with an interrupted employment record or periods of part-time work since the final pension was to be based on the uprated value of earnings over the 'best twenty years' of an employee's working life. It allowed some years of low pay or absence to be discounted. Part-timers were covered, provided that they earned enough to trigger National Insurance contributions: the hope was that most people would realize at least twenty years of full-time earnings.

Employers had to offer men and women 'equal access' to occupational pension schemes: men and women in the same category of jobs were to be equally eligible. But the license to include or exclude employees by 'occupational group' meant that far more men than women were contracted out of SERPS. It continued to be legal to exclude part-timers: most did not qualify for membership of an employer's pension scheme, even in the public sector. The mandatory provision of pension for widows confirmed a trend towards increased pension provision for survivors which was showing up clearly by the early 1970s. Widows of men in SERPS could add their late husband's pension entitlements to their own, provided that the total did not exceed the maximum single person's pension. All members of contracted-out occupational pension schemes were guaranteed benefits at least as good as those they would have received had they remained in SERPS. All state pensions in payment were to be index-linked in line with which ever was the greater—annual retail price or annual pay increases. By this time, virtually all contracted-out occupational pension schemes were based on final salary levels, which, again, offered some hedge against inflation (Groves, 1983; 1987).

However, the 1975 provisions introduced by a Labour government with all party consent, after many years of debate and failed legislation, were unexpectedly short-lived. A Conservative administration passed the Social Security Act 1986. From the end of the century, SERPS benefits will be severely downgraded. From 1988 employees have been able to opt out of SERPS or an occupational scheme in favour of a new 'personal pension' scheme that permits people to build up their own individual pension funds, to which employers are not required to contribute. The 1986 legislation does not affect women who have already retired, whose financial circumstances are addressed in the next section. The changes will undoubtedly have a potentially more dramatic effect on the future pension entitlements of younger women than on that generation of older women who will be retiring from paid work before the end of the century (Groves, 1991).

Income, poverty and the current generation of retired women

Research carried out in the late 1950s and early 1960s revealed substantial income poverty among elderly people (and elderly women in particular) and provided impetus for pension reforms in the 1970s. As today, those people with occupational pensions were demonstrably less at risk to poverty, although a small employer's pension in some cases merely meant that people were not able to claim means-tested social assistance, rather than that they were better off. Few married women had an employer's pension in their own right. It was a minority of women (mainly teachers or other public-sector workers) with such pensions, and most were single. The many widows whose husbands' employment had conferred no occupational pension rights were substantially at risk to poverty, as were any 'lone' women who lived on into 'old' old age (Groves, 1987).

By the early 1980s it was still the case that such lone elderly women were at risk to poverty, with 80 per cent of all lone female pensioners over 60 living 'on the margins of poverty' with incomes of not more than 140 per cent of the then means-tested supplementary benefit rate (Walker, 1987). Around two-thirds of all men were in poverty, married or single. A government survey of 1982 (DHSS, 1984) showed that, as before, receipt of an occupational pension was the key to living above the poverty line in retirement; that men were far more likely than women to have employers' pensions; and that men's pensions were of more value than those of women. The most recent information concerning elderly women's incomes is from analysis of the GHS of 1985 and 1986 by Sara Arber and Jay Ginn (1991a). Among people over 65, men (62 per cent) were far more likely than women (25 per cent) to have an occupational pension. Married couples were far more likely to have occupational pension income than lone women, with divorced women the least-favoured. Older men tended to be less well off than younger men, whereas women's incomes in retirement varied far less with age. However, non-state pension income (the crucial factor in lifting individuals out of poverty) showed a large gender difference, with 50 per cent of men but only 20 per cent of women receiving more than £5 per week, and 26 per cent of men and a miniscule 7 per cent of women more than £25 per week. The top 10 per cent of men were receiving over £60 per week in all non-state income whereas the top 10 per cent of women received over £16 (p.382). Some interesting questions can be raised as to the relative extent of poverty and deprivation among married and lone women.

Some other 'markers' as to the extent of poverty among retired women include numbers claiming means-tested income support, with 1 147 000 women claimants over pensionable age in 1989 and a further 118 000 couples over 65 (DSS, 1991b). It is known that a proportion of pensioners do not claim their social security benefits: in 1986 it was estimated that 21 per cent of pensioners were not taking up their entitlement in full (Hansard, 1986). Early research on the take-up of loans from the Social Fund also appears to indicate that elderly people are significantly underrepresented among applicants (Gillian Stewart and John Stewart, 1991).

It has to be said that there has been virtually no research into the particular income position of older women from black and minority ethnic groups. Given their small number, even large national sample surveys have not produced sufficient data to enable analysis by race (Arber and Ginn, 1991a). Evidence from employment histories cited earlier would lead us to conclude that they are as vulnerable, if not more so, to poverty as older white women. Certainly many will have had too few years in employment to earn a full state pension or, because of their low-paid unskilled work, to benefit from an occupational pension. Moreover, those older women primarily from the Asian communities who came to the UK as elderly dependents are reliant on financial sponsorship and have no entitlement to state pensions or benefits (Fenton, 1987). For them, financial dependence is likely to be most acute.

Older women and occupational pensions

Given the very small amounts of many occupational pensions, mere receipt of an occupational pension does not of itself guarantee freedom from financial want. Payment of a lump sum by the pension fund at the time of an employee's retirement may place the recipient above the capital limit set for receipt of means-tested benefits. Only later, when the capital has been drawn upon or has eroded in value, will the pensioner actually become a potential income-support 'statistic'. Furthermore, remembering the limitations of defining poverty on a 'poverty line', there must be many pensioners who, while not technically in poverty as defined by eligibility for means-tested benefits, are none the less

living in financially modest circumstances which preclude full participation in activities or the enjoyment of goods and services available
to the majority of people in control of an earned or more substantial
retirement income. Women in particular, with their interrupted work
records and tendency to earn less than their male counterparts, even
in the better types of full-time employment, are at risk to ending up
with modest occupational pensions.

In addition, occupational pensions can lose their value over time.
Public-sector pensions are currently uprated in line with prices,
although in the 1970s they were (like state retirement pensions during
the same period) uprated in line with whichever was the greater
rise between earnings and prices. Private-sector pensions are not
automatically increased: their value depends only partly on government regulation and they are subject to decisions as to what the
pension fund can afford. Women, who have longer life expectancy
than men, are particularly affected by erosion of pensions and capital
in old age. It has been estimated that during the 1980s a single pensioner lost £11.75 and a couple £18.95 on the value of their state
retirement pension alone (Oppenheim, 1990).

When Mrs Gillian Shepherd announced in Parliament, 2 July 1990,
that 70 per cent of the recently retired have occupational pensions,
85 per cent have income from savings, while half own their own
homes, the response must surely be to ask—how much pension, how
much in savings, and is the home ownership an asset or a financial
burden? And how, in particular, do the figures relate to elderly
women? Pensioners on low incomes (among whom women are over-
represented) are vulnerable to the 'poverty trap'. A pensioner on
income support (plus housing benefit and community-charge relief)
may be little or no worse off than another pensioner whose occupational pension simply cancels out any entitlement to means-tested
benefits.

To reiterate, while it is hard to get detailed figures on elderly
women's incomes and we know even less about how fairly incomes
are shared in married households, it is clear that among the present
retired population it is women with a substantial record of full-time
public-sector employment who are likely to be best off in terms of a
fully index-linked employer's pension. Single women are most likely
to have a full National Insurance pension earned in their own right.
Married women, to date, have very limited entitlement to occupational pension benefits in their own right, since many have spent long
periods in non-pensionable employment (including part-time work)
or out of the labour market. Women widowed during their husband's
retirement lose household income, in that they typically get half of
their husband's pension as a widow's pension. However, there are
still many widows whose husbands were never in an employer's pension scheme: the husbands themselves may have had inadequate

occupational or state pension records due to unemployment, changing jobs, illness or working abroad. There is also very little known about women's access to capital and the extent to which women themselves generate wealth in their own right or inherit money from people other than their husbands. It is to be hoped that women's separate taxation will, in due course, allow information on women's individual wealth to be compiled.

The major factor which has depleted women's incomes in old age compared with men's is unpaid work. Compounding this has been the reluctance of employers to admit women to occupational pension schemes, the concentration of women around poorly paid, part-time occupations, lack of career advancement (so that women have ended their working lives with lower pay than their male contemporaries) and the fact that the current generation of elderly women was normally required by their employers to retire at 60, whereas a majority of men have been permitted to work on until 65. Benefits for widows were designed to compensate for loss of a husband's income. One of the major problematic areas of pension provision in the more recent past has been that pension providers have steadfastly equated 'doing something for women' with improving widows' benefits, thus reinforcing financial dependency in marriage rather than enabling women to defer their earnings in their own right. A high marriage rate in the post Second World War era allowed employers increasingly to discount the pension needs of independent women who were, by definition, 'older' single women. In future, problems of pension entitlement will be compounded by a higher divorce rate and the fact that single women will quite commonly have borne children and, for this reason, taken time out from the labour market.

The present generation of retired women, especially the younger ones with a near-universal marriage rate, have been exceptionally dependent on their husbands for their financial welfare in old age and pension provision has been organized on this assumption. Those retired women who have been living entirely on state National Insurance and means-tested benefits have done badly in the past ten years. This generation of older women is not, in general, well off on its own individual pension contributions and investments. As Jane Falkingham and Christina Victor (1991) show, there are few 'woopies' among them. Are the older women now in their fifties likely to have fared better?

The 1990s: older women, paid work and future poverty

A key question is whether the current generation of women in their fifties is likely to be substantially better off than previous generations in old age, the result of pension and retirement benefits earned in their own right. This seems unlikely. Their access to a state retirement pension in their own right will be limited, despite the 'credit' system for household responsibilities. Older women's membership of occupational pension schemes is associated with lengthy full-time employment and higher pay (OPCS, 1990d). Again, most women now in their fifties do not fulfil the conditions for entitlement.

The over-fifties have not been a 'high-flying' generation as far as paid work is concerned, although they have certainly been economically active. In 1980, when in their forties, nearly 80 per cent were in paid work, although around half worked part-time. On average, they had spent around eleven years outside the labour force since leaving full-time education. Those in their later forties had put in twenty years of paid work, of which over five had been part-time (Martin and Roberts, 1984). This generation moved into its fifties in the 1980s. Wells (1989) has pinpointed their economic activity between 1984 and 1987 when the worst effects of the economic recession of the early 1980s were beginning to lift. Around two-thirds of women in their early fifties were economically active and half of those in their later fifties, evenly split between full and part-time work. Women have tended to stop paid work before reaching pensionable age (Martin and Roberts, 1984). Parker (1980) found that the 'stayers' were full-timers or those whose part-time jobs were 'main life work', while most (87 per cent) female early retirers lived in households with another earner. Obviously those women who are earning pension entitlements have a major incentive to stay on until 60.

Wells' (1989) analysis of the 1984–1987 Labour Force Surveys (UK) showed that women in their fifties were employed in very narrow sectors of the labour market—clerical (38 per cent), personal service (30 per cent) and professional (16 per cent)—whereas older men were 'spread across most occupations'. This is not a well-qualified generation and it is one whose schooling was substantially disrupted by war and its aftermath. In 1987, of the 55–59 age cohort, only 7 per cent of women had degrees or professional qualifications and 64 per cent had no qualifications (Wells, 1989). The majority left school before 16, and had no access to schooling which led to formal qualifications. This general lack of qualifications is one factor which has put this generation of women at a disadvantage in their working lives, barred them from obtaining better paid jobs and put them at particular risk to unemployment. It is also the case that many women, however well qualified, have experienced downward occupational mobility upon returning to paid work after a break, especially when the return was part-time (Martin and Roberts, 1984). The difficulties experienced by highly qualified women (now over fifty) who were attempting to hold down 'top jobs' in the 1970s has been discussed in detail by Fogarty *et al.* (1980).

Women's low earnings are also problematic in terms of making financial provision for old age. In 1990, even full-time, non-manual women in their fifties were earning on average only £221 per week compared with £383 for men: only 10 per cent of women earned more than £337 (Department of Employment, 1990, Part A, Table 13). Only 10 per cent of *all* women were earning more than £200 per week (Department of Employment, 1990, Part E, Table 124), and part-timers were particularly low paid, with only 12 per cent of saleswomen or shop assistants earning more than £4 per hour and only 4 per cent of nursing and midwifery (NHS) staff earning more than £10 (Department of Employment, 1990, Part F, Table 171). In this situation it seems unlikely that most women can do much to enhance their pension entitlements. Women members of an occupational pension scheme can sometimes pay additional voluntary contributions (AVCs), although this facility is rare outside the public sector or nationalized industry schemes (Sue Ward, 1990). If an older woman can buy in 'added years' and use them to increase the total number of completed years of service counted in a pensions scheme related to 'final salary', this can be an excellent way of boosting pension entitlements. Where an employer does not offer such a facility, women in late middle age (like men) are faced with the problem that buying free standing AVCs or any type of personal pension from a commercial provider involves paying much more than would be the case for a younger purchaser and the commission charged can be expensive (Ward, 1990).

There are also issues relating to women actually being able to keep their jobs in late middle age. Anne Harrop (1990) comments that most studies of older women over the past two decades show that they experience considerable social and economic disadvantages compared with older men or younger women. In 1990, prior to major recession, there was much publicity in the media around efforts to encourage older workers to return to or remain in the labour market, and to this end the 'earnings limit' applied to retirement pensioners was abolished in 1990, permitting state pensions to be drawn regardless of continuing earnings. In June 1991 the government announced that the whole issue of equalizing pensionable ages for men and women in state and occupation pension schemes is to be reviewed, leaving open the question whether women's notional 'working years' are to be extended, or men's shortened (*Guardian*, 1991). Meanwhile, in the 1980s full-time women workers in permanent jobs with occupational pension benefits have been (like men) encouraged to take early retirement with enhanced pensions. This includes that minority of well-qualified women (mainly teachers) over 50 who are currently being targeted for 'voluntary redundancy'. Other older women will lose their jobs and have difficulty in finding others, not only due to shortage of jobs but on account of prejudice against older workers. Jane Straw (1990) notes that 'Prejudice against older people rests . . . on the belief that certain skills and abilities have been lost, without being replaced by other qualities' (p.8). Apart from the fact that skills are not necessarily atrophied through age, such prejudice against older workers weakens their position when management is seeking to cut costs by 'losing' older (and in some cases better paid) workers.

Harrop (1990) argues that 'Employment practices that favour younger workers and encourage older workers to take early retirement weaken the position of older workers in the labour force' (p.8). Women in hierarchical occupations such as teaching, within which women have, to date, had restricted opportunities for career advancement, are particularly at risk to being labelled as 'unsuccessful' and ripe for early retirement if they have not advanced, by their fifties, to a point to which men typically advance. In some occupations, 'youthful' looks are preferred for women staff. Married women with adult children and whose husbands are in full-time employment are still subject to the familiar accusation of not 'needing' a job.

Most women now in their fifties are, if in paid work, concentrated in the low-paying service sectors, with one in two female employees working part-time. Most earn modest wages or salaries, are less likely than men to be in a pension scheme, have put in fewer years than men (in general) in schemes and have had less opportunities to accumulate savings. In any case, as has been pointed out, for this generation it has been seen as a husband's place to provide for old age. Among the women most likely to be heading for poverty in retirement, and especially if they live a long time, are married women whose husbands themselves have generated inadequate retirement/widows' benefits (often through illness and unemployment); single women with a lifetime of low pay behind them; divorced or separated women who have lost a 'family wage' and potential widow's benefits from a husband's earnings; and any single women who (less commonly in this generation) had children and brought them up on their own.

All too little is known about the economic activity of women in their fifties or about the problems which older women face in the labour market. Privatization of public-sector employment can downgrade service conditions and threaten pension rights. There is little doubt that 'life-cycle events that exclude women at certain stages of their lives in the formal labour market commit them to a financially disadvantaged position at older ages' (Harrop, 1990). As Shirley Dex and Chris Phillipson (1986) argue: 'Few of the reforms aimed at women have achieved success in the crucial area of job security and pension provision in middle and later life. An extensive debate and analysis of the rights of older women is now urgently required' (p.82).

Conclusion

This chapter has focused on the financial circumstances of the current generation of older women. It has shown that older women, with their characteristically interrupted employment careers, financial dependence in marriage and low earnings have limited potential for experiencing the 'Third Age' outlined by Laslett (1989) as a period of 'leisure, independence and education'. 'Few, or very few of the large numbers of British wives, widows and spinsters who since the 1950s have lived long enough . . . have been in a position' to afford a Third Age lifestyle. Thus, 'the principles and ideas of Third Age living are a mockery for the poorer old, who have been and lamentably still are, so large a proportion of those in retirement' (p.91).

The present generation of retirement pensioners, and especially women, are best served by social policies which ensure adequate income and a dignified way of life, including fully indexed state and occupational pensions, good public services and general concessions for elderly people. This means cheap housing and utilities, good low-cost public transport, and access to education/leisure facilities and health/social services which are free at the point of delivery. Where the majority of elderly people have to live on modest incomes, as in the UK, they need collectively provided and publicly subsidized services. Merely targeting means-tested benefits at the poorest pensioners is a highly questionable strategy (Vanessa Fry *et al.*, 1990).

During the 1980s, government policies have emphasized the desirability for individuals to make provision for their own old age, notably by means of personal pensions, but nowhere have the implications for women been spelt out (Groves, 1991; Davies and Ward, 1992). It is necessary to consider how, in future, younger generations of women might be helped to make better provision for their own old age. With a high divorce rate, this is a necessity.

Policies which enable women to build up entitlement to a full state retirement pension by means of contributions and credits are an essential foundation for adequate income in old age, provided that the level of that pension is itself adequate. It can be argued that such a basic pension should be available as a citizen's right and funded from taxation (Midwinter, 1985). The original SERPS scheme was the best second-tier provision yet devised for women who do not have access to a good occupational pension scheme. It recognized problems of absence from the labour force and fluctuating earnings by basing the eventual pension on a contributor's 'best twenty years'. There is no reason why a future government should not devise a replacement which could match the best occupational schemes and obviate the problem of people moving between jobs. Personal pensions are meant to deal with the latter problem, but they are problematic for women who tend to take 'time out' just when contributions should be paid in full for maximum benefit and who typically have periods of part-time work (Davies and Ward, 1992).

Meanwhile trade unions have a part to play in encouraging employers to offer good occupational pension schemes with coverage of lower paid workers. It is important that, as far as possible, women can make up missing contributions and work on through their fifties, should they so desire. Under European Community law, all rules of entitlement for pensions of any kind will in due course have to be sex-neutral (Davidson, 1990), and it will be important that any potential disadvantages for women during the period of adjustment are monitored. It will also be important to continue monitoring the impact on women of the new 'personal pension' arrangements. Much more information is needed on the impact on women of changes in pension provision over recent decades.

Much still needs to be done to raise women's consciousness with regard to the complexity of pension provisions so that they do not, for instance, fail to join a good employer's pension scheme (as is now permitted) and instead choose a personal pension scheme offering potentially inferior benefits. However, it is the unequal division of labour in the home which prevents many women from being more financially independent: good childcare provision and carers' services would help. Given the high divorce rate and the fact that a proportion of women do not wish to marry, and leaving aside issues of financial equity in marriage, good arguments can be made for all women to have the option to be economically self-sufficient. This self-sufficiency must extend into old age. It can be argued that until then women will not be full citizens (Ruth Lister, 1990). The women's movement needs to give more attention to issues relating to older women, and it is to be hoped that in the future older people in general will become a far more potent political force. At the present time we appear to be moving towards even greater economic inequalities between individuals in old age, with women at the bottom of the heap.

4 Health issues and the older woman

Moyra Sidell

'. . . We've always been walkers. We still are. We still walk quite, well, seven or eight miles now. We used to walk a lot further when we were younger . . . I've had rheumatism and arthritis since I was in my twenties. But I mean my legs were all right. And we proved it, we used to walk ever such a lot . . .'

(Ray)

Introduction

Health is not a simple concept. It is difficult to define and consequently difficult to measure. In 1955 the World Health Organization defined health as, 'not merely the absence of disease and infirmity but complete physical, mental and social wellbeing'. Despite this, the traditional way to measure the 'health' of a society, or a group within it, has been to take statistics on mortality and morbidity as indicators of health. When these criteria for measuring health are used, the outcome for older people can be summed up in Constance Nathanson's (1977) phrase: 'women get sick, but men die'.

Concentrating on death and disease is a very negative way of accounting for health: it tells us nothing of people's subjective experiences or of health in a more positive sense. In the case of older women, it also reaffirms the negative stereotyping to which they are subjected and which depicts them as decrepit and a burden on the nation's resources. It takes no account of their differences in relation to age, class or ethnicity. Nor does it acknowledge the many older women who are without disease or disability. However, the dilemma we face is that in trying to counter these ageist attitudes, we may unwittingly minimize the health problems with which some elderly women have to contend. The sprightly senior citizen can be a very oppressive role model for someone coping with the pain and immobility of arthritis. Therefore, in any discussion of the health of older women, it is important to acknowledge the very real health problems they face without reinforcing ageist attitudes.

Some of the tension between positive and negative interpretations of the health status of older women lies in the nature of the available evidence. 'Objective' measures, which monitor disease and disability, present a negative picture of the health of older women. But, statistics relate to populations, whether national, regional or on the basis of some other grouping: they never describe the experience of individual people. They are useful in indicating overall areas of concern and can help target resources. They can tell us the probability levels of disease and disability. But to understand how older women experience health we also need to explore their subjective accounts and find out how they interpret this difficult concept.

This chapter draws on a study of gender differences in the health of older people (Moyra Sidell, 1991). It combines, or triangulates, three types of data to try to understand better the complex issue of the health status of older women (Leonie Kellaher *et al.*, 1990). First, national data sets on mortality and morbidity were used to provide measures of disease and disability. This was followed by secondary analysis of large-scale sample surveys to explore self-reported illness, use of services, assessments of health, and health beliefs and attitudes. Third, biographical interviews with thirty individual older women from a range of backgrounds were conducted, to provide insights into how health is subjectively experienced.

In comparing three such data sets, the contradictions are immediately exposed. Mortality and morbidity statistics tell us that women live longer than men, but in so doing they accumulate a range of degenerative diseases which are not necessarily life-threatening but are likely to be highly symptomatic. Yet the subjective evidence on self-rating of health tells us that a significant number of older women assess their health as good in the face of this 'objective' evidence of the coexistence of disease and disability. All this begs the question as to how individuals interpret the concept of health: we cannot assume a shared understanding.

We therefore begin this chapter by examining the self-assessments of health made by older women. We then go on to look at the ways in which the health of older women is measured, exploring the many contradictory findings which exist. Finally, we ask if, and why, our existing healthcare system fails them, and raise a number of issues about improving the health status of older women: issues which are developed further in Chapter 9.

What is health?

Self-assessments, beliefs and attitudes

In assessing their own health elderly people are an anomalous group (Cox *et al.*, 1987; Christina Victor, 1987). For all other age groups, measures of self-assessed health correlate well with 'objective' measures of ill health. A large proportion of older people, however, rate their health as 'good' or 'fairly good' in spite of suffering from some form of chronic disease or disability. Older women too seem to have a fairly optimistic view of their health. The GHS 1985 (OPCS, 1987a) found that only 25 per cent of older women assessed their health as poor, 37 per cent thought it was fairly good and 38 per cent good. Yet the GHS also reports that 60 per cent of all women over 65 are suffering from a long-standing illness or disability.

Older men and women are even more optimistic when asked to rate their own health in comparison with their peers (Cockerham *et al.*, 1983). Such positive assessments have been attributed to two factors. First, the fact that they have survived into old age puts them in a 'healthy' category. The second factor is more practical, and suggests that because older people do not have to maintain a high level of functioning their health is 'good enough' to meet their needs. However, even when they think that their own health is reasonably good, there is evidence that they still feel vulnerable and worry about becoming a burden to others. This comment from a 72-year-old woman in the biographical study was typical:

'I think the deep-seated anxiety is, am I going to become incontinent, dotty, not able to communicate, and a burden?'

Generally too, the women I interviewed played down their health problems. They would typically say, 'Oh I'm fine in myself, it's just this . . . stiff knee/high blood pressure/trouble with my water-works . . .' Clearly then, many women are assessing their health not just in terms of the presence or absence of disease, or in terms of function; they feel well in spite of their illness or disability. We therefore need to understand what it is that people mean by 'health'.

The Health and Lifestyles Survey (HALS) by Cox *et al.* (1987) asked respondents what it felt like when they were healthy. Well over half of men and women between the ages of 64 and 75 expressed their health in terms of feeling good. But this was less so for the very elderly men and women who were more inclined to think of health in terms of being able to function adequately. What was also clear from the biographical interviews was that health encompasses a range of physical and emotional elements. It is certainly not a one-dimensional concept but ranges from physical and functional elements, through emotional, psychological and spiritual dimensions. Jessie, a 67-year-old West Indian woman, described it in these terms:

'Well, I think good health is when you can laugh and make people laugh. People say that riches is money, but riches is when you can laugh and make somebody happy.'

Strength too was very much a feature of good health, while weakness was associated with ill health. There was also a marked tendency for health to be seen as personal responsibility. To admit to ill health is to admit to being weak and unwholesome. This coincides with the findings of Jocelyn Cornwell (1984) and Clare Wenger (1988), who found that their respondents were reluctant to admit publicly to ill health:

'Good health is associated with right attitudes and moral fibre and complaining and talking about health problems is seen as self-indulgent' (Wenger, 1988, pp.12–13).

There are also differing cultural concepts of health and disease. Many people from eastern cultures, in common with white Anglo-Saxons, believe that health means 'having no illness'. However, because of their religious beliefs they may perceive disease to be more the result of God's punishment or the environment than of infection or the malfunctioning of the body (Qureshi, 1991). An in-depth study by Jenny Donovan (1986) of attitudes and beliefs about health and illness amongst Asian and Afro-Caribbean people of all ages provides us with additional material about the experience of health and wellbeing of older black and minority ethnic women. Many of her respondents felt that life in the UK was unhealthy. The cold damp climate, the lack of fresh food and experiences of racism and loneliness led to depression, illness and worry. This compared unfavourably with the much 'healthier' lives they felt they had left behind and which they associated with warmth, friendship, abundant sunshine and fresh food.

Whether these views were realistic is not the point. What is at issue is the fact that they were having to adjust to a way of life which for them was less than satisfactory. Older people generally have to make a great many adjustments (Coleman, 1990b), some minor, some major such as retirement or the loss of a spouse. It is also important to recognize that people whose backgrounds and origins are different from where they live out their later years are likely to have greater adjustments to contend with.

Health and wellbeing then is dependent on a complex set of social, psychological and physical factors. The interaction of chronic illness and disability with other influences such as the existence of intimate relationships with family or friends, the ability to pursue interests or hobbies, as well as the material conditions of their lives, will affect how individuals experience and therefore assess their own 'health'. It would also seem that good health is not incompatible with illness or morbidity, issues we now consider in more detail.

Mortality, illness and morbidity

If we take longevity as a measure of health, then it is clear that ever since the start of mortality record keeping in 1841 women have lived longer than men (see pp.2–3). The difference has gradually widened until the 1980s when signs that the gap may be stabilizing or even getting narrower are beginning to emerge. So, in terms of mortality, women are 'healthier' than men.

The precise reasons for women's greater longevity are unclear. Suggestions include: gender-linked physical differences; different responses to environmental hazards; different health habits, for example smoking and drinking; personality differences—men are said to be more aggressive and willing to take risks; and differences in reactions to illness and disability, with chronic conditions being diagnosed earlier (Ingrid Waldron, 1976; 1982). In terms of reactions to illness and disability, all the literature on self-reported illness claims that women report more illness than men and that this is maintained into older ages, with elderly women frequently reporting multiple illnesses (Lois Verbrugge, 1984; 1985; Helen Evers, 1985; Myrna Lewis, 1985; Victor, 1987).

The HALS (Cox *et al.*, 1987) records the prevalence of symptoms reported by respondents in the past month. Table 4.1 indicates that substantial minorities of older men and women experience various symptoms. However, with the exception of ear trouble, kidney and bladder trouble, coughs, and flu/colds, women report a good deal more symptom than do men.

As well as these physical symptoms, the HALS records symptoms of mental malaise. Here the differences between older men and women are even more marked, as Table 4.2 shows. Again, women report more problems in all categories. Yet, although many more older women than older men are subsequently diagnosed by their GPs to be suffering from mental illness, proportionately more older men are hospitalized for this condition (DHSS, 1989; RCGP/OPCS and the DHSS, 1986). While one would not wish more older women to be admitted to mental illness hospitals, the evidence suggests that older women's mental symptoms are not treated as 'seriously' as older men's but they are nevertheless labelled as 'mentally ill'.

In addition, whilst our knowledge about mental health in old age is limited and patchy, it is possible to distinguish between conditions which affect all age groups and those which are specific to elderly

Table 4.1   Prevalence reported during the past month of selected physical symptoms.

	Reported (per cent)	
	Women over 65 (n = 936)	Men over 65 (n = 697)
Painful joints	45	30
Eye trouble	31	18
Bad back	29	18
Palpitations	29	24
Foot trouble	28	18
Flu/colds	26	26
Headaches	24	13
Stomach trouble	23	19
Ear trouble	19	21
Sinus trouble	17	16
Constipation	16	11
Faints	14	8
Cough	11	14
Kidney and bladder trouble	8	8

Source: Cox *et al.*, 1987.

Table 4.2   Prevalence reported during the past month of selected mental symptoms.

	Reported (per cent)	
	Women over 65 (n = 936)	Men over 65 (n = 697)
Difficulty sleeping	41	23
Worry	28	11
Always tired	26	17
Difficulty concentrating	17	11
Suffers from nerves	17	6
Feels lonely	14	10
Feels bored	13	11
Feels under strain	6	4

Source: Cox *et al.*, 1987.

people (Victor, 1991). There is, for example, little evidence from the mental malaise index referred to above that older people suffer any significantly higher rates of symptoms than do younger people. However, this is not the case for conditions such as dementia. Several types of dementia exist (Jorm *et al.*, 1987), but there are considerable difficulties associated with accurate diagnosis and assessment. This is particularly so in the early stages, and in instances where there might be language deterioration and communication problems with members of black and minority ethnic groups and bilingual clients (Deidre Duncan, 1991; Clephane Hume, 1991). Such difficulties have led to quite marked discrepancies in both the prevalence and incidence figures across different studies (Carole Brayne and David Ames, 1988). This is compounded by the fact that studies have often used different research tools and different ways of collecting and defining their information, so that the data we do have can only be regarded as an approximate guide (Victor, 1991).

Despite these methodological problems, current evidence suggests that the prevalence of dementia 'is about 1 per cent for the population aged 65–74 and 10 per cent for those aged 75+' (Victor, 1991, p.93). We also know that dementia occurs more frequently with increasing age, and some recent studies contend that women are two to three times more likely to be affected than men (Copeland *et al.*, 1987; Morgan *et al.*, 1987; Vetter *et al.*, 1986). Senile dementia of the Alzheimer's type is also thought to be more common in women (Jorm *et al.*, 1987). Once again however, it is important to note that in all cases we are dealing here with minorities of older people.

Further 'objective' evidence about the health of older women comes from measures of the incidence of disease and disability. To obtain a picture of the morbidity of a live population, there are two useful sources: the Hospital Inpatient Enquiry (DHSS, 1987) and the Morbidity Statistics from General Practice (RCGP/OPCS and the DHSS, 1986). These two sources show that for older women, as well as men, diseases of the heart and circulatory system predominate. Within this category, minorities of women suffer from hypertension and other non-life-threatening forms of circulatory diseases such as phlebitis and varicose veins. There are considerable differences between minority ethnic groups and the indigenous population. Coronary heart disease, for example, is much more prevalent amongst South Asian men and women, whereas hypertension and strokes are more common within the Afro-Caribbean community. Malignancies are high on the list for men and women but, whereas up until the age of 65 women have higher rates of cancer, particularly of the reproductive system, after the age of 65 men predominate, particularly with cancer of the respiratory system. We also know that elders from black and minority ethnic groups are afflicted by these conditions too (Bennett and Ebrahim, 1992). The other notable disease category which affects older women is that of the musculo-skeletal system, including the non-life-threatening diseases such as osteo- and rheumatoid arthritis and osteoporosis. All are highly symptomatic.

Older women also feature in the Hospital Inpatient figures through accidents, injury and poisoning. Broken bones, particularly fractured femurs, account for a high proportion of the admissions of older women, and clearly osteoporosis is an important factor here. However, a league table of risk to osteoporosis shows up the variations between different ethnic groups: Northern white women and Asian women are most at risk; Hispanic, Mediterranean and Jewish women are in the middle; and Afro-Caribbean women are least at risk.

Fractures in older people are not only attributable to osteoporosis. We know that some older people are prone to falling; women more so than men. Smith (1992) links this to a number of factors including hypothermia, the overprescribing of tranquillizers, and drugs given to lower blood pressure which make some people feel dizzy. Bruises and lacerations, which are also unusually high for women over the age of 75, could also be due to the adverse effects of prescribed medication. In fact, most of the 'poisoning' which affects older women is due to prescribed drugs, both correctly and incorrectly administered. For example, it is estimated that up to 80 per cent of women over the age of 75 are taking at least one prescribed medication, and that much of this treatment is unnecessary and unwarranted (Burns and Phillipson, 1986; Bennett and Ebrahim, 1992). Older people are particularly at risk to adverse reactions, to excessive prescribing and to poor supervision of long-term medication (Bennett and Ebrahim, 1992). In the absence of alternative therapies or preventative measures, many are overreliant on things such as sleeping pills and are afraid of trying to manage without.

A striking feature of the morbidity of women in later life is the existence of these non-life-threatening but highly symptomatic conditions. In order to assess the impact of these conditions, we can turn to two further sources of information: the GHS (OPCS, 1987a) provides data on the incidence of chronic illness and disability in the non-institutionalized population, while the OPCS disability survey (Jean Martin et al., 1988) provides information on the whole population. This is important when investigating the health of those over 75, as the most frail are likely to be in hospital or residential homes (Victor, 1991).

The OPCS study reveals that 63 per cent of women in the age group 65–74 have a long-standing illness compared with 60 per cent of men. This increases with age to 73 per cent of women over the age of 75, and 69 per cent of men. In her discussion of these figures, Christina Victor (1991) cautions us not to be too pessimistic, pointing out that not all those with a long-standing illness or disability are restricted in their activities. However, we must also remember that chronic conditions such as arthritis are long-term health problems, and that the term 'disability' has many and varied dimensions. We know too that the prevalence rate of different types of disability increases consistently with increasing age and that older women are more likely to experience chronic ill health than are older men

(Martin *et al.*, 1988; Verbrugge, 1989). More specifically, we can explore the notion of 'disability' further by considering the different ways in which women and men may be incapacitated in later life.

Studies which examine older people's ability to function or undertake what are commonly termed 'Activities of Daily Living' reveal that the vast majority are able to get around outside their own homes, perform basic self-care tasks, and engage in activities such as shopping and cooking, unaided. Sara Arber and Jay Ginn (1991c), in their recent analysis of GHS data, show that in many categories women are likely to report being more impaired than men. For example, over the age of 65 they are twice as likely to report impaired mobility. Moreover, using a measure of overall disability, very elderly women are particularly disadvantaged: over the age of 80, nearly 25 per cent of women are 'severely' disabled compared with 11 per cent of men. One consequence of the degree to which older women suffer from functional disability is that they may well require both more informal (see p.113) and more statutory care.

There are however problems inherent in either overstating or understate the level of disability in the population of older women. If we overstate the case, we reinforce the negative stereotyping of older women and encourage lower expectations of health. If we understate the levels of illness and focus on fit and well older women, we do a disservice to those who are suffering from chronic conditions. The pressure is then back on them to minimize their difficulties and to look for remedies in themselves, rather than making legitimate demands on the health services.

Older women and their doctors

One particularly crucial element of our health services is of course the GP. The gender differences identified above in relation to reports of illness, and morbidity and functional disability, are also evident when we look at patterns of consultation. Research shows us that women of all ages consult their doctors more than men. Although the gap between men and women narrows with age, older women make up a substantial proportion of GP consultations. Roos and Shapiro (1981) also found that a small number of elderly people use the services a great deal, while data from the National Morbidity Statistics for General Practice (RCGP/OPCS and the DHSS, 1986) shows that only one-quarter of women over 65 had not consulted their doctor at all in the year prior to the survey. Consultation patterns also vary according to social class, marital status and housing situation. The GHS (OPCS, 1987a), for example, shows that widowed women, those from social classes IV and V, and council-house tenants, are amongst the highest consulters of doctors. We also know from Ken Blakemore's work (1982) that high proportions of elderly Asians and Afro-Caribbeans visit their GP.

Blakemore (1982) has suggested that for immigrants from ex-colonial countries, the family doctor service was a familiar, although scarce, resource. Black and minority ethnic older people therefore value and use the service when it is freely available. This is one of the things which makes residence in the UK worthwhile when set against many other disadvantages.

In considering these consultation patterns, we are faced with yet another paradox. While objective statistical data shows us that women consult more than men, evidence from qualitative studies suggests that women are in fact extremely reluctant to visit their doctors (Mildred Blaxter and Eric Patterson, 1982). This was certainly the case with the older women who participated in the biographical study. The overwhelming impression was that one should not bother the doctor unless absolutely necessary. This almost amounted to a moral code and many talked of putting off seeing the doctor until absolutely necessary. Typical was one woman who, at 94 years of age, said:

> 'I only call the doctor when I'm forced to, when I really do feel ill. I had diarrhoea once everso bad, and this here warden, she would call the doctor. I say, what, for the diarrhoea. But I'd had it everso bad, about three weeks. That was the warden what done it, that wasn't me.'

Or another woman, who remarked:

> 'I always put it off—I say it will go, or I can cope with it, and put it off until suddenly I say, you bloody fool, you'd better go and see him. He can't bite your head off. I don't like going to doctors. I don't like the whole experience.'

None of the women took the decision to visit their doctors, or to call him or her out, lightly. And however much time they had on their hands, a visit to the doctor was not seen as a diversion. Their reluctance to 'bother' the doctor was due to a variety of reasons. Some showed extreme respect for the doctor's time; others were frightened of what the doctor might tell them. But many felt that their complaints were not of sufficient magnitude to take to a doctor or, that on past experience, the doctor would have no answer to their problems.

Explanations of the health status of older women

Why is it then that older women report more symptoms of illness, consult their doctors more, and are said to be suffering from more medically diagnosed mental and physical illness than older men? Biological and physiological evidence is only part of the picture. A great deal of the difference can be explained by reference to the social environment and women's roles throughout the life course (Lewis, 1985).

In their review of the literature, Ellen Gee and Meredith Kimball (1987) discuss various explanatory models, including three which imply that women's illnesses are not 'real', and that the differences we see between men and women are due mainly to women's willing-ness and opportunity to report illness. The 'role compatibility' model for example, suggests that women's roles are not so demanding as men's roles, therefore it is 'easier' for them to be sick (Nathanson, 1975). This is closely related to the 'fixed role obligation' model (Marcus and Seeman, 1981), which asserts that women have fewer role obligations that cannot be changed, and thus are freer than men to be ill. The third, the 'social acceptability' model (Phillips and Segal, 1969), argues that women are given 'cultural permission' to be sick and that:

'therefore, women feel less constrained than men to define and report mild symptoms as illness and to adopt the sick role' (Gee and Kimball, 1987, p.34).

These three explanations assume that men and women experience the same level of symptomatology, while a fourth model (Gove and Hughes, 1979) attempts to explain why women experience higher levels of symptomatology and more 'real' illness than men. The authors claim that women's nurturant roles are in fact so demanding that the attendant stresses lead to 'real' illness. Later, Gove (1984) linked this to the 'role obligation' model, arguing that it was also easier for women to adopt the sick role and admit to these 'real' illnesses.

There are many problems with all these models. In particular, they fail to differentiate between women in terms of age, class, race, sexual orientation, marital status or employment status. Role obligations for example, might be quite different under these varying circum-stances, and differentially affect women's opportunities to go sick. Moreover, as Christina Victor (1991) notes: 'It seems likely that sev-eral factors account for the gender differences in morbidity and that there are different explanations for different types of illness' (p.74). This interaction of factors is evident in a condition such as depression. In younger women, depression has been specifically linked with the housewife and mother roles (Ann Oakley, 1976; George Brown and Tyrril Harris, 1978). However, poor physical health and adverse life events such as loss, and particularly loss due to bereavement, are also associated with depression in older women (Elaine Murphy, 1988). In the USA too, Himmelfarb (1984) has found that housing quality, social support and undesirable life events, particularly bereavements, are all correlated with women's mental health. While the evidence is clear that women in general, and older women in particular, report more symptoms of a psychological nature than do men, it is the translation of this 'mental malaise' into medically diagnosed mental illness which is disturbing.

By definition, a medical diagnosis such as depression is made by a medical professional, and much of the statistical evidence we have on gender differences in morbidity is processed by members of this profession. Consequently, it is important to consider just what part they themselves might have to play in explaining older women's higher rates of morbidity relative to men. There is now a great deal of evidence which suggests that the still male-dominated medical profession perceives its male and female patients differently. For example, one GP in Helen Roberts' (1985) study of women and their doctors says this:

> 'For women, perhaps 50% of their complaints are psychosomatic; for men, perhaps 30% would have a psychosomatic side to a physical complaint—for instance, a duodenal ulcer' (p.40).

It is interesting that the GP qualifies and legitimizes the male psychosomatic complaints. Helen Roberts also draws on evidence from medical textbooks, medical training, and interviews with medical practitioners, to show that the GP quoted above was by no means untypical. Jacqueline Wallen (1979) has also concluded that:

> 'The doctors studied were more likely to see their female patients' illnesses as psychologically caused and were more pessimistic about their recovery' (p.145).

Clearly, sex-role stereotyping affects the clinical judgement of some doctors.

In the National Morbidity Statistics for General Practice (RCGP/OPCS and the DHSS, 1986), GPs are also asked to rate the seriousness of consultations. Here we discover that a higher proportion of women's consultations are considered 'trivial' than are men's, although the gender differences are less marked at older ages. The use of the terms 'serious' and 'trivial' are themselves misleading, adding to the impression that women consult their doctors unnecessarily. In fact, in National Morbidity Statistics for General Practice, the terms 'serious' and 'trivial' mainly refer to the degree to which a condition is life-threatening. But, as we have seen, a good deal of women's complaints in old age are not so much life-threatening as highly symptomatic, and would therefore only qualify for the epithet 'trivial'.

In discussing health issues and older women, it is apparent that we are faced with a number of paradoxes. First, they live longer than men but, in so doing, they are more likely to be afflicted by a variety of chronic conditions. Second, although the 'objective' data tells us that many older women are affected by highly symptomatic conditions, subjective evidence reveals that they generally assess their own health as good. Third, more older women than men consult their doctors but, for a variety of reasons, they are extremely reluctant to do so. These paradoxes call into question the appropriateness of our existing healthcare system in meeting the needs of older women.

Enhancing the health of older women

In the light of their beliefs and attitudes about health, we need to ask what can be done to help older women to 'feel good' and to function well. What does the medical profession have to offer in terms of treatment and cure? What is the role and scope of self-health care, health education and health promotion, and what preventative measures are likely to affect future generations of older women?

In order to enhance the health of older women there are a number of key issues which have to be considered and tackled at a variety of levels, from the individual through to the organizations and institutions which make up our healthcare system. In the remainder of this chapter we shall focus on five areas:

• research and information
• self-healthcare
• professional attitudes
• life-enhancing care
• health promotion and prevention

Research and information

To counter either an overly negative or an overly positive stereotype, it is necessary to break down the existing statistical data into recognizable chunks. As we have seen in the introductory chapter, the category 'older woman' spans at least thirty years: it includes women who are currently married; women who have never been married; and women who are widowed, divorced or separated; it includes women who have and have not borne children; those who have operated in the public world of paid employment; and those who have spent most of their lives engaged in domestic work. As well as these dimensions there are differences of class, sexual orientation and ethnicity.

Whether we use objective or subjective measures of health, the argument that age acts as a 'leveller' in terms of social inequalities is not borne out. Data on marital status is one example. Measured both objectively and subjectively, the health status of widowed women is poorer than that of women who are married or single. In terms of medically diagnosed disease and disability, married women are in better health than single older women, although single older women report fewer symptoms and assess their own health as more positive than their married or widowed counterparts. Single older women seem more robust and to have a better sense of wellbeing than either married or widowed women (Sidell, 1991). Class has also been shown to have a similar significant influence on the health status of older women. Arber and Ginn (1991c) report evidence of a five-year 'class gap', indicating that 'in each age group, unskilled women are more likely to be disabled than higher middle-class women who are five years their senior' (p.124).

Aside from the necessity of analysing existing data in more detail, it is also important to address areas where there is a marked lack of information. In particular, there is a lack of research on the health of older lesbians and black and minority ethnic older women. For older black women however, we can begin to piece together a picture of their health situations from a number of studies (Blakemore, 1982; Barker, 1984a; Bruce Holland and Gillian Levando-Hundt, 1987), while a number of writers have summarized the very few epidemiological differences which emerge (Alison Norman, 1985; Bennett and Ebrahim, 1992). However, culturally insensitive remedies, together with racist and sexist attitudes, compound the difficulties which black and minority ethnic older women face in relation to obtaining the health services they need. Graham Fennell and his colleagues (1988) make this point well:

'In thinking about health and illness of older Asians and Afro-Caribbeans, it is clear that "exotic" illnesses of ethnic minorities are a very small part of the issue. More important are the trends in illness resulting from social disadvantage: poverty, poor housing and environment, compounded by racist assumptions and ethnocentric service organizations which fail both to inform themselves about culture and health needs of ethnic minorities, and to respond appropriately' (p.133).

Although the health problems experienced by black and minority ethnic older people are largely similar to those of the indigenous population, they face what Alison Norman (1985) has described as the 'triple jeopardy' of age discrimination, socio-economic disadvantage, and discrimination in access to services because of culture, language or religious affiliation. These are formidable obstacles although, as we see below, gaining access to formal services is only one element in the complex process of enhancing the health of older women.

Self-healthcare

In the maintenance of health and wellbeing, self-health care practices are crucial. Professional health services, contrary to popular opinion, actually play a very small part. In addition, the ideas and concepts involved in self-health care are not new: older women have long practised such behaviours in relation to both their own health, and that of their families (Cornwell, 1984). Self-healthcare has been defined by the World Health Organization as:

'all the actions that an individual takes to prevent, diagnose, and treat personal ill health; all individual behaviours calculated to maintain and improve health, and decisions to access and use both informal support systems and formal medical services' (Coppard *et al.*, 1984, p.3).

It also includes decisions to do nothing (Kathryn Dean, 1986). At an individual level, the most common self-healthcare practice is self-medication. In addition, with growing information about the various effects of such lifestyle factors as nutrition and exercise on health and well-being, older people too are becoming increasingly involved in a range of health-related activities (Miriam Bernard, 1985).

However, Kathryn Dean (1982) has shown that older people's health knowledge and basic treatment skills are poor, despite the fact that many of these skills are relatively easy to teach (Coppard *et al.*, 1984). In a review of self-healthcare and older people carried out for the World Health Organization (Coppard *et al.*, 1984), five such skills or components were identified:

- simple diagnostic skills—which the individual might use to estimate her health status, e.g. breast self-examination, monitoring pulse rate, checking temperature
- skills relevant to simple acute conditions—including treatment of the common cold and everyday illnesses, and first-aid for non life-threatening conditions
- skills needed to treat chronic illness—such as self-monitoring and following prescribed regimens
- skills for disease prevention and health promotion—including exercise, diet, avoiding tobacco and alcohol abuse, good dental hygiene and healthy lifestyles
- health information skills—such as what steps to take prior to seeking professional treatment, how to obtain health information and how to gain access to formal care

Despite a growing number of developments in Europe and North America which address these different skills, together with an increasing amount of research (Cynthia Savo, 1984; Dean *et al.*, 1986; Social Science and Medicine, 1989), British work in these areas is very patchy and limited. Unfortunately, as Jocelyn Cornwell (1989) has observed: 'Health professionals have on the whole left it to community groups and voluntary organisations to satisfy the health education needs of elderly people and carers' (p.10).

Examples of the kinds of self-healthcare developments which have occurred in this country in recent years can be found in the Age Well Ideas Packs produced by the (then) Health Education Council and Age Concern. More particularly, the work of Pensioners Link in London, and of The Beth Johnson Foundation in Stoke-on-Trent, has shown that there is potential and scope for enhancing the health skills of older women through a variety of means such as health courses and talks, activities and exercise, easily accessible health information and advice, and through peer support (Bernard, 1988; 1989; Miriam Bernard and Vera Ivers, 1986; Kathy Meade, 1986; 1987; Ivers and Meade, 1991). While an overt aim of such developments is to impart a sense of self-determination to older women and to encourage more positive images of old age, it is not intended that they should replace formal services. In fact, self-healthcare and professional care are complementary systems. Rather than being outside the remit of health professionals, there is no reason why such initiatives could not be facilitated by medical and nursing staff, given appropriate gerontological training (Chris Phillipson and Pat Strang, 1986; Bernard and Phillipson, 1991).

Professional attitudes

In their dealings with health professionals, it is evident that older women have to contend with a number of difficulties, in particular the giving and receiving of information, and the ageist manner in which they are often treated. This may well compound the sexist and racist treatment meted out to them. Older women's encounters with their doctors can be less than satisfactory; as the Waterloo Pensioners' Health Group (Action for Health, 1988) explains:

> 'We get the feeling from our GPs that we have been here too long, that we are too old for treatment. We know we do get aches and pains but it's not necessarily our age. For anyone of any age, something can be done.'

The women in the biographical study also objected to being told that their condition was to do with their age. Many of the chronic conditions that afflict older women, such as arthritis, do not respond to a medical model of treatment and cure, and so threaten the competence of the doctor. By putting it down to age, the doctor is able to shift the responsibility back onto the individual, reinforcing the negative stereotyping which older women so often meet. They are made to feel guilty for bothering the doctor and to have very low expectations of getting relief from their symptoms, which is often what they want most of all. Older women also feel that they are not listened to and that the doctor is not interested in their version of things. As one woman said to me:

> 'I've lived with this body for 70-odd years now. If I don't know when it's not working properly, I don't know who does?' (Quoted in Sidell, 1992).

Nor are they given enough information by their doctors as to what is wrong with them, why they are being prescribed a particular form of treatment or drug, and what to expect from it. As well as medication for high blood pressure, older women are frequently prescribed psychotropic drugs, especially tranquillizers and antidepressants. Many of the interviewees were unhappy with this, and felt that writing a prescription was a way of avoiding a lengthy consultation. As one woman said:

> 'He'd write the prescription out as if he wanted me to hurry up and get out' (Quoted in Sidell, 1992).

Others went to their doctors in times of stress, particularly after a bereavement, and instead of the emotional support that they were seeking they were given tranquillizers or sleeping pills. One woman went to her doctor after her husband died because she felt 'bad'. She said:

> 'He just gave me sleeping pills. I don't know what they were. I was dead scared to take them. I just came out, and that was it. When I got home, I didn't take them, I just got better on my own' (Quoted in Sidell, 1992).

As we saw above, non-compliance with treatment and taking medication incorrectly are problematic. Much of this could be avoided if older women were given satisfactory explanations by their doctors. This is crucial because older women are particularly dependent on their GPs to help them cope with some of the disadvantages they face, especially in extreme old age (Arber and Ginn, 1991c). Frequently they feel disappointed and dissatisfied with the treatment they receive. Health professionals of all kinds should also be alert to the different cultural concepts of health and disease held by their older patients, and be considerate of the rituals they may practice in relation to health maintenance (Qureshi, 1991; Arlene Trim, 1992). Unfortunately however, the training of many health professionals fails to include transcultural health care (Trim, 1992), one result being that existing services are often insensitive to the needs of ethnic older people (Bennett and Ebrahim, 1992). Nor, as we noted above, does it adopt a gerontological perspective, despite the fact that there is now some evidence that ageist attitudes amongst health professionals can be effectively countered through students having contact with well, older people in mutual learning situations (Aldeman *et al.*, 1988).

However, the real problem lies not with a handful of GPs whose manner leaves a lot to be desired, but with a discriminatory and ageist system of healthcare which still focuses largely on cure, with perfunctory attempts at prevention. For many older women their condition is not amenable to cure and it may be too late for preventative measures to be effective. What they require is symptom relief in its widest sense, with attention paid to the social and psychological as well as the physical aspects.

Life-enhancing care

Despite the comments made above about the curative model of healthcare, it is important to acknowledge that there are a number of successes of medical science which can radically affect the health, wellbeing and quality of life of older women. Joint replacement is one such intervention. A graphic illustration comes from a woman in the biographical study who was 64 when she developed osteoarthritis, first in her right hip and then in her left. She was on the waiting list for a hip replacement for four years before being operated on.

Before her hips were bad she was extremely active; a keen bowls player and a member of various clubs. She went regularly on camping holidays with her nephew and niece but, as the pain became greater, she became immobile and had to give up all her activities. She described what it was like to get about before the operations:

> 'I used to get off the bus down the road and how I walked up here! . . . I used to look round, Oh God, please let me get home, you know. That was dreadful. It was frightening just going to put one foot down and drag the other along. I kept looking round to see if anyone was watching me, you know. That was awful, that was. Nobody knows, well they do, those who suffer with it.'

For a year she lived on painkillers and was more or less housebound. But, after two operations in the space of eighteen months, she felt as fit and healthy as she had ever done and was looking forward to going camping with her relatives.

Another woman had been waiting for two years to have an operation on her knee. Although apprehensive about the surgery, she was keen to have it done because she and her husband lived in a first-floor council flat and she felt she would be unable to manage the stairs for much longer. She had been told that if she was prepared to go privately, she could have the operation immediately, but the £3000 required was way beyond her means. When every year is precious, and when deterioration of the joint and possible damage to the surrounding muscle tissue, combined with a gradual lowering of morale due to constant pain, threaten the success of the operation, it seems to make little sense to delay these operations for even months let alone years. Yet, most people face years of misery waiting not for a life-saving operation but for a life-enhancing one.

In the case of joint problems it is the political will to provide the resources for these life-enhancing operations, not the inadequacy of modern medicine which is the problem. The present generation of older women have been nourished on the promises of the NHS and naturally turn to their GP when in need. Most have neither the means nor the inclination to seek help in other quarters, and consequently have come to accept very low expectations of any improvement in whatever condition may be affecting their health and wellbeing.

The chronic illnesses and negative life events which many women experience as they age, detract from their sense of wellbeing. Opportunities for 'feeling good', contented and happy can be threatened by pain, discomfort, loneliness, grief, anxiety and loss of self-confidence. Palliative care and symptom control, pioneered by the hospice movement, offers one possible way forward. The basic principles of such life-enhancing care centre around the relief of symptoms, whether they be physical, social, psychological or spiritual. However, most GPs do not possess an appropriate range of skills. Yet, counselling, physiotherapy, occupational therapy, as well as complementary therapies such as acupuncture, massage and aromatherapy, could all provide relief without some of the adverse side effects of prescribed medicines. The need to treat, cure and relieve symptoms is vital for those who suffer from chronic illness and disability. But what scope exists for preventing illness and promoting good health?

Health promotion and prevention

The scope for detecting and preventing illness and disease amongst older people is a problematic issue. Melanie Henwood (1990a) for example, argues that older women are discriminated against in many screening campaigns. They are either left out altogether or are not sufficiently well targetted. For instance, although 40 per cent of deaths from cervical cancer occur in women over 65, Department of Health guidelines specifically exclude screening or regular follow-up of women over this age (Henwood, 1990a). It has also been suggested that screening and case-finding for osteoporosis would be cost-effective and save much distress and loss of life (Henwood, 1990a). Various measures such as Hormone Replacement Therapy (HRT) are now available to counteract some of the more debilitating effects of the menopause from which some older women suffer, and to help in preventing osteoporosis. Screening procedures would therefore make good sense. However, many women understandably feel ambivalent about the use of HRT. Evidence about its effectiveness and its safety remains conflicting and confusing. If HRT can alleviate some problems and prevent others from developing in the future, then we should not be prejudiced against its use. But, women need unbiased information in order to help them make choices about whether or not it is appropriate for their own situation. Nor should its use preclude an exploration of other methods of alleviating some of the stresses which occur at the time of the menopause.

More generally though, screening procedures have been found to be of doubtful value, and can be intrusive and generate feelings of anxiety unless used with a great deal of sensitivity (Freer, 1985; Taylor *et al.*, 1983). Jane Tilston and Jude Williams (1992) distinguish between screening and case-finding, defining the latter as 'identifying those people at risk of losing their ability to function independently' (p.208). The new GP contract makes provision for just this type of intervention, requiring GPs to make annual contact with all their patients over the age of 75. At these consultations they should check on mobility, general physical conditions and the use of medication. They are also required to take account of the social environment. In theory, this comprehensive check allows for the identification of a range of needs, but it is a matter of concern that the increased work-load may discourage GPs from taking people over 75 onto their lists. This would have serious implications for older women.

One approach which seems more appropriate to this type of needs assessment is the use of biographical interviews such as those developed by Tim Dant and his colleagues (1989) in their research with Gloucester Health Authority. Trained 'care coordinators' under-took these interviews in the homes of very frail elderly people. The 'holistic' view of health which they obtained enabled them to contex-tualize current health needs in the past and present social, economic and psychological environment of the elderly person. Articulating their own health needs in this way, rather than passively accepting a 'package' of available services, is important to help maintain independence, prevent deterioration and generally to improve wellbeing.

Improving health and wellbeing can also be achieved through health education and promotion. The difficulty with much existing work in this area however is that it is aimed at the individual. On the one hand it appeals, in that it aims to give individuals some control over their own health; on the other hand, it makes them responsible for their own health and can so easily lead to 'victim blaming'. It also diverts attention away from structural causes of ill health such as poor housing, lack of education, and poverty.

Aggregate problems require aggregate measures. Hypothermia is a case in point. Many older women live in a state of 'fuel poverty': they have little to spend on heating and often have the hardest houses to heat (Stella Lowry, 1991). In addition, older people are more likely than younger people to be at home all day, and so need to heat their dwelling constantly. The policy response to the threat of widespread hypothermia in very cold weather has been to individualize the problem. As Lowry (1991) says:

> 'Even the campaigns to prevent hypothermia have degenerated into an obsession with individual behaviour: stay in one room, wear several layers of clothes, and knit yourself a woolly hat' (p.12).

There are a whole range of other public policy issues which affect the health of older women. Campaigns to improve public transport, the fight for decent pensions and realistic extra heating allowances, are as much a part of health promotion as posters urging individuals to eat more fibre than fat. Health promotion thus has to operate at both the societal level and the individual level if it is to be effective in improving the lot of older women. All too often the political will to tackle issues such as poverty and poor housing is lacking, whereas it costs little to urge people to exercise.

Conclusion: the future health of older women

Some older women live till their late eighties and early nineties and remain fit and disease-free. Others will suffer from physical or mental, chronic, debilitating illness for many years. Yet others have periods of chronic illness and periods of fitness. The permutations are many and varied. Trying to predict whether the patterns of health and illness we currently see will remain in the future is very difficult and, as yet, it is unclear whether lengthening life expectancy will mean improving or worsening health for older women.

This issue has led to vigorous debate in gerontological circles since James Fries (1980) first proposed his 'compression of morbidity' thesis. He argued that as mortality was reduced and, as people lived longer, the onset of disability would be delayed. Changes in life style and in individual behaviour, through things like giving up smoking, taking regular exercise and eating a healthy diet, would also be influential (Fries, 1980). The result would be that the period during which people were sick and incapacitated would become compressed into the few years before death.

This optimistic view has been reviewed and challenged by a number of authors (Bury, 1988; Manton, 1982; Verbrugge, 1984; McKinlay *et al.*, 1989). Given our present considerations, it is also important to note that Fries' thesis may in fact have more salience for the lives of men than for women. Older women, as we have seen, are much more likely to experience non-life-threatening chronic conditions and, as Arber and Ginn (1991c) show, a comparison of disability rates between 1980 and 1985 reveals little evidence of improvement in their conditions. For example, there was hardly any change at all for women over the age of 80, compared with a fall of almost 10 per cent in the proportion of men of the same age who were severely disabled.

This debate highlights the need for us to look closely at what we know about the health of women in later life. Paying attention to diversity in their health status is vital if we are not to stereotype older women's experiences either negatively or positively. But, in so doing we must guard against individualizing the health difficulties that some older women face. Many of their health problems stem from structural factors such as poverty and social class (Arber and Ginn, 1991c), and are not within the individual's control.

In terms of healthcare provision, our healthcare system still operates on a treatment and cure basis and fails to provide relief from the unpleasant symptoms of some non-life-threatening, chronic conditions. But if 'health' is truly to represent anything other than just the absence of disease, and if we are really concerned with promoting the wellbeing of older women, then the central question we have continually to demand an answer to is: 'How can we get older women's health concerns taken seriously without over-medicalizing them and taking them out of the control of women themselves?'

5 Intimacy and sexuality amongst older women

Dorothy Jerrome

'. . . I made life-long friends. We all did. You know with the girls. And they've all since married, got families, they're grandparents now. And the men, we made friends with the men. I mean, we went out with the men sometimes. And for company . . . and as I say one of my friends has now been in Canada for many years, and I always did fancy going to see her, but never had the chance. Anyway she had a stroke now and can't write. Her husband writes at Christmas . . . And Jessie was bridesmaid to a friend in Newcastle . . . And the last time we saw her she'd been in hospital sixteen years and all she could do was move her head . . . and she knew we were coming, she'd got all the old battery photographs out, and we took ours . . .'

(Ray)

Introduction

The lives of older women express many themes in common with their younger sisters: the search for intimacy, coming to terms with physical changes and the demands of the body, fulfilment of personal potential. The search for intimacy may be conducted in different settings as family constellations change and new personal needs become apparent.

In this chapter we shall examine the range of relationships which give purpose and meaning to the lives of older women. The family, as representing an area of major emotional investment, is a suitable starting point. We shall consider the changing experience of women as mothers, daughters, sisters, grandmothers and granddaughters, and as partners. The role of wife and experience of marriage is one most women share, although for many older women it is a thing of the past. The subject of widowhood provides a bridge to a discussion of loneliness and the significance of intimacy in women's lives. We then explore the importance of friendship and peer relationships.

Lesbianism, as a sexual orientation and a special kind of friendship, occupies the remainder of the chapter.

Women in the changing family

The impact of demographic changes on family structures has been substantial. The consequences for women of historical depth, the shorter distance between the generations, the ageing of the family, and its structural complexity, are far-reaching. The family represents an area of major investment. Outliving their male partners who tend to be married until they die, married women form closer relationships with female kin up and down the generations (Gunhilde Hagestad, 1985a). Younger generations more often have contact with old women than old men in their families. The oldest family member known to children as they are growing up is likely to be a woman.

Women are, in any case, the kin-keepers, those family members who take responsibility for keeping track of personal developments and sustaining links between the generations and between the different branches (Carolyn Rosenthal, 1985). It is the women in the middle generations who are most frequently allotted this role, although the lines of communication run through women in all generations (Rosser and Harris, 1965). Women bring families together. They organize the get-togethers, remember the birthdays, and write the festive cards, often to their husbands' families as well as to their own (Hagestad, 1985a). Importantly, this function is common to most cultures even if the activities are different.

The role of 'family monitor' extends to the giving of care and support, an issue which is taken up in the following chapter. For the present, we need to note that the older woman's position in the multigenerational family creates both challenges and difficulties by virtue of her kin-keeping role. As a result of their substantial investment in other people's lives, women often mention events that happened to other family members when asked to describe good and bad things that have happened to them. The evidence suggests that, 'especially in the case of stressful events, this vicarious involvement in the "ups and downs" of others may leave women with a sense of powerlessness and overload' (Hagestad, 1985a, p.149).

Some of the strain comes from the lack of certainty about appropriate ways of behaving in the contemporary situation of the multigenerational family. Rights and obligations may not be so clearly defined and, in the absence of role models, some women may be vulnerable to excessive demands. Hagestad quotes studies which identify the plight of the young–old woman on whom the burden of care for both older and younger kin falls. A strong sense of jealousy sometimes occurs in those older women who feel they are denied the privileges of old age because even older women receive all the attention. In minority ethnic communities, there may be tensions between generations of women who are caught by the cultural expectations of their country of origin and the changed conditions in the UK. Even without such negative consequences, the ambiguity of terms and roles inherited from an earlier family system is problematic. Hagestad provides an example of a family gathering in which a child cried 'grandma', and three women, from three generations, responded. Confusion exists in other areas, too. There are few prescriptions for behaviour between step-relations, and cultural developments (the liberation movements of the 1960s and 1970s and patterns of migration, for example) have introduced uncertainty into relationships between spouses and between middle-aged parents and their adult children. Family relationships for the dominant culture in the UK have always offered scope for negotiation, in the absence of clear prescriptions for behaviour (Dorothy Jerrome, 1990b). In the multigenerational family of the late twentieth century, however, there is a need for innovation, and new conflicts of interest may be settled in ways experienced as stressful and unfair by some of its female members. New freedoms for some mean new constraints for others.

Women across the generations

Mothers and daughters

Although the propensity to marry has increased so that more older women are likely to have become wives, parenthood is by no means a universal experience (see pp.113–14). It is even less likely, given the decline in family size, that a woman will have had a daughter. Evidence from the 1971 Census (OPCS, 1983a) indicates that the average woman marrying in 1945 at the age of 24 would, at the age of 50, have borne on average just over two children. As many as 37 per cent would have either no children (10 per cent) or only one child (27 per cent). Using these figures as a basis for prediction, we can assume that in the years leading up to the turn of the century, over half of very-aged women will have either one or no living children (Timaeus, 1986). These findings put into perspective the earlier ones of Abrams (1978) which used to seem astonishing: that in the late 1970s over one-third of elderly people (over 75) had no children. The statistics in those days were offered to place in perspective the popular and professional view that elderly women living alone were being neglected by their adult children. The evidence today is provided with the same end in view: to alert policy makers to the likely future needs of very-old women (Gibson, 1990).

Looking at the transactions that go on between the generations, we need to examine various popular and professional assumptions. One is that older members are dependent on younger; another—the empty-nest syndrome—suggests that women in midlife are heavily dependent on their growing children for a *raison d'etre*. Both assumptions imply an imbalance, with women presented as vulnerable and inferior.

Recent evidence suggests that, contrary to the popular stereotype, the flow of family resources is not all in one direction, with the old woman being the principal beneficiary. Dependency within the family is now understood in terms of the history of interaction between its members. A system is not suddenly invented as a member develops new needs (Lewis, 1990; Kuypers and Bengtson, 1990). At each stage of the family cycle we can observe dependency in excess of culturally sanctioned levels: the young adult who continues to depend on middle-aged parents; the parent who prolongs a sick role longer than is necessary. But the direction of dependency—older on younger or *vice versa*—is not a forgone conclusion.

It is easy to assume that an old woman lives with her adult daughter to be cared for by her. However, as Clare Wenger (1992b) points out, such arrangements are generally set up before the need for care emerges, and it is difficult to say who is dependent on whom. The relationship of mothers and daughters is built on a lifetime of reciprocal exchanges (Wenger, 1992b; Hagestad, 1985a; Jerrome, 1990b). Reciprocity has taken over from 'filial responsibility' as a key concept in intergenerational relationships in the 1980s.

Women in the middle generations are likely to be caught up in servicing the needs of both younger and older kin. They might expect to enjoy the rewards of their earlier investments in care when they themselves are old, but might not receive them. A benefit women anticipate with near certainty in western culture is the departure of adult children. It used to be assumed that women who had devoted themselves to caring for their families would find themselves facing new feelings of anxiety and depression with the loss of a major role—the empty-nest syndrome. This notion persists in some quarters. In fact, many women do not feel this way. The reduction in day-to-day mothering tasks is generally anticipated with pleasure and a sense of a life task successfully accomplished (Gemma O'Connor, 1988). The self-concept is often more positive when the responsibilities of day-to-day child-rearing are removed (Marilyn Block *et al.*, 1981; Margaret Huyck, 1989). Women who view the departure of children with mixed feelings, or for whom the 'loss' is experienced as stressful, are in the minority.

The phenomenon of the empty-nest syndrome used to appear in the literature alongside the concept of the 'postparental' phase of life. The notion that mothering stops at the point of children's departure from the family home is unhelpful. Women do not stop being mothers, although the quality of mothering may change. They enjoy a new freedom to be themselves, although financial constraints and restricted job opportunities limit the capacity for full autonomy. The menopause, which often coincides with the departure of adult children, is no longer viewed as a kind of death, but a release to enjoy many years of active life. Frustrations arise less from the loss of fertility than from the pressures of caring, and lack of money.

There are certain situations today which threaten cultural expectations of retirement from active mothering in midlife. Unemployment and housing difficulties mean that adult children are staying longer in the family home. The lack of independent living opportunities and support services for disabled adults makes it even more problematic for them to leave home. The rise in divorce may also place pressure on mothers in particular—given the strength of female ties mentioned earlier, coupled with the tendency for women to gain custody—to provide not only emotional but also housing, financial and childcare support to adult daughters.

The likelihood of older women entering into this latter relationship with their daughters and grandchildren depends on a variety of factors. A woman's health and employment status will affect her availability and capacity to care. So will her ideas about such issues as rights and responsibilities in marriage. Changing ideologies of family life and child-rearing over the past fifty years can generate conflict between mothers and daughters (Jerrome, 1990b). One of the things parents strive for is continuity: indicators in the behaviour of their children that they have managed to transmit what is best in their own lives (Bengtson, 1989; Coleman and MacCulloch, 1985; Marjorie Fiske and David Chiriboga, 1985). A child's divorce and in particular a daughter's bid for independence, can threaten this continuity. Whatever she feels about her daughter's actions, however, the elderly mother will often respond positively to the needs of the grandchildren.

The discussion so far refers mainly to elderly white women. Less is recorded about mother–adult daughter relationships in black and minority ethnic communities. Concepts of dependency and interdependency between generations have different implications for the lives of minority ethnic older people and their families. In Asian cultures, for example, dependency on adult children is traditionally viewed more positively, as natural and healthy as is the continuing involvement of older adults in their adult children's lives. Within this context, older women derive status from their continuing role in the domestic sphere sustaining relationships both within and between households. But this extended family structure with its accompanying roles and obligations has, like the nuclear family, been subject to change. First-generation elderly women from minority ethnic communities may experience alienation from their second-generation daughters or daughters-in-law who have been influenced more strongly by British culture (Margaret Clark, 1969; Glendenning, 1983). In many West Indian families, the uncertainty of relationships between mothers and daughters may be due to the latter having been left in the care of grandmothers in the Caribbean. For other older women who may speak little English and for whom there are few opportunities to develop new social networks outside the family, the positive aspects of the 'empty nest' experienced by white women may not be available. Other frustrations are due in large part to the inadequacy of space, poor accommodation and the isolation resulting from family members being out at work or at school all day. While increasing numbers have adopted a more nuclear living situation, proportionately more West Indian women still live with younger people than their elderly white counterparts, at least in inner-city areas (Blakemore, 1983a), and a significant number of Asian older people live with their children and grandchildren (Liam J. Donaldson and Aileen Odell, 1984).

Grandmothers

Within the contemporary western family structure, the role of the grandmother is vague and undefined. There is enormous variability in its performance. This is hardly surprising, given the tendency for grandchildren to be any age between newborn and 60, and grand-parenthood to occur from about 30 until old age (Hagestad, 1985b). The average age to become a grandmother in the UK today is in one's fifties (Sarah Cunningham-Burley, 1985). This is a time when a woman is likely to be in paid employment and leading an active lifestyle. In the late twentieth century lifespan the onset of this role, and its duration, mean that traditional images of grandparenting are often out of date (Featherstone and Hepworth, 1989). The traditional media image, embodied in the Queen Mother—'the universal Grand-mother'—no longer fits the practice.

The contemporary image is positive, although some women still find it difficult to reconcile this with their self-image as active and youthful. A radical lesbian grandmother talks of the contradictions her new status creates for her, particularly when her grandchild is male and the experience of being a grandmother cannot easily be discussed with childless lesbian friends (Marcy Adelman, 1986). A range of styles is evident in contemporary grandparenting: formal; funseeking; distant; remote; companionate; and involved. Grand-mothers behave differently over time and with different grand-children (Karen Roberto, 1990; Thompson *et al.*, 1990).

In many black and minority ethnic communities, the grandmother role is more formally constructed within the extended family network. In the West Indian family for example, grandmothers have been expected to play an active part in childcare, often enabling their daughters to work. With greater numbers of mid-life and older women now involved in the labour market this role is having to be renegotiated. In the Chinese and Asian communities, grandmothers also play a significant role in maintaining cultural identity and keeping their grandchildren in touch with their mother tongue and customs.

On the negative side, divorce reminds us that grandparenthood is contingent on the actions of other people. It is adult children who produce the grandchildren and control access to them. The most vulnerable relationship in divorce is said to be between a man and his son's children, given that women have normally been awarded custody. An older woman is more likely to keep in touch with her divorced daughter-in-law, as 'the mother of my grandchildren'. Under the 1989 Children Act grandmothers can remain centrally involved in the welfare of their grandchildren following divorce. The act empowers them to apply to the court for a share of parental responsibility and they are recognized as parties to divorce proceedings concerning children.

Family contemporaries

Within the family, lateral ties are also important to women. Sisters and cousins, husbands and brothers form part of the supportive network. Research on sibling relationships has proliferated in recent years in the USA, although not in the UK (Victoria Bedford and Deborah Gold, 1989). It is justified partly by the demographic trends which make groups of siblings ageing together an increasing likelihood. Ties between brothers and sisters rest on shared family history, on long-term commitment and on peer-group membership. Closeness rests less on frequency of contact than on memories of a shared past (Jean Scott, 1990). As they age, siblings grow more accepting and approving of one another. The death of parents is a time when the sharing of activities and sense of similarity increases. A large number of old people identify at least one sibling as a close friend.

Sisters tend to be closer than brothers. They provide each other with a range of benefits, such as companionship, housing in widowhood, and social stimulation through shared activities like shopping and attending club meetings.

The death of a sibling affects an old woman's sense of vulnerability and identity. The loss of the sister who has been a best friend and co-resident can precipitate affective disorders such as depression and anorexia. An old woman encountered during my research on clubs had stopped eating on the death of her sister. It had coincided with the installation of the brand-new kitchen they had planned together.

The kitchen remained as bare and unused as on the day of her sister's death. As possibly the longest intimate tie experienced by women, and one which can potentially meet every need apart from physical intimacy, the importance of sibling relationships needs to be recognized.

More is known about elderly sisters than brothers, partly because they are more numerous. Many questions remain unanswered, however. One, which will be addressed in the following chapter, concerns their role as care-givers. How do siblings collectively respond to parental needs? Which sibling is nominated to care, and why? Sibling rivalry, much studied in children, remains unexplored in old age, although Margaret Forster's recent novel 'Have the Men had Enough?' (1989) begins to touch on these issues. Carried over from early to late life, sibling rivalry can be exacerbated by parental preference or rejection, which may extend to dead as well as live children. Aged parents may reverse their preferences in the absence of the favoured son or daughter in order to acquire the necessary support (Sam Moss and Miriam Moss, 1989). We might imagine the pleasure or bitterness produced by such shifts in allegiance.

Marriage

Compared with old people no longer with partners, married couples live longer, stay healthier and feel better, although in each case the relative advantage for men is greater than for women (Jessie Bernard, 1973; Beth Hess and Beth Soldo, 1985). In general there are, for demographic reasons, increasing numbers of long-term marriages. Despite the rise in divorce rates that increase the likelihood of women entering retirement alone, the number who are still with their husbands after fifty years has grown (Gibson, 1990). Variations among ethnic groups may need to be borne in mind although little data are available. There is some evidence that West Indian women, for example, are less likely to enter retirement with a husband, for reasons including lower male life expectancy and lower rates of marriage (Blakemore, 1983a).

Evidence of golden wedding couples suggests a special quality of intimacy and satisfaction (Brubaker, 1985). However, we should not minimize the existence of conflict in later-life marriages. Studies of marital satisfaction suggest a series of peaks and troughs over the life course, although the methodological basis of such work limits its usefulness in relation to old age (Jerrome, 1990b; Walker, 1977). Those marriages that survive may give a false impression of contentment. The longer the relationship, the more salient it is to self-identity and the harder to disengage from, or admit to failure. It is also possible that couples whose marriages have survived fifty years have remained married because their expectations have been scaled down to fit existing possibilities. The very negative status associated with divorce may have also contributed to the survival of marriages within the current cohort of older women. Until the last twenty years only a very small percentage of women experienced divorce. It was not unusual for them to pass themselves off as widows or to revert to their original names if childless.

Intactness, therefore, is not by itself evidence of marital satisfaction (see p. 158). Indeed, the majority of stable relationships might be far from the vital and fulfilling ideal celebrated in popular culture. From the conflict-habituated relationship described in fiction (Simenon, 1972), to the ideal partnership which these days graces the front covers of retirement magazines, a range of types exists. The retirement of one or both partners, and the impact of catastrophic illness (Kuypers and Bengtson, 1990), can profoundly affect the relationship. Adult children also have a role. Their involvement in problematic late-life decisions where couples disagree is powerfully demonstrated in Tillie Olsen's fictional account 'Tell Me a Riddle' (1980). In this case an old woman's deep wish to savour the emptiness of the family home, where she has always before had to 'move to the rhythms of others', is thwarted.

Remaining single

There are misconceptions about the social needs of some groups of older women. The never-married, for example, are popularly assumed to be lonely and bitter. In fact, the lives of single women, one of the most stereotyped groups, display themes similar to those of their married counterparts—the centrality of family relations and the development of close personal relationships over time (Katherine Allen, 1989). Unlike some widowed and divorced women, the single older woman seems to benefit from a lifetime of coping socially and emotionally, in a society which values coupledom and where marriage and parenthood are seen as signs of maturity and normality.

The increasing propensity over the century to marry makes older single women a diminishing category. The demographic factors—an imbalance of men and women, and the tendency for men to choose younger wives—which kept many women single in earlier decades —is less likely to affect future cohorts. However, it would be misleading to suggest that all older women would have married if they could. Many remained single through choice, for career reasons or to care for elderly relatives. It is also the case that women from higher socio-economic classes have shown a greater propensity to stay single.

Sexuality

Studies of sexuality in later life are, like those of marital satisfaction, difficult to pursue (Jerrome, 1990b). However, it is now well known that, contrary to popular assumption, older people are sexual beings. The benefits of physical intimacy continue to be enjoyed by women with healthy partners until extreme old age, although the pattern reflects earlier rates of activity. In some cases sexual activity ceases relatively early, but this is often the culmination of an unsatisfactory relationship. Some women feel with the arrival of the menopause that they can legitimately give up an unrewarding activity. More often it is husbands who are responsible for the termination of sexual activity, through ill health or impotence caused by temporary disability or fear of failure. Social attitudes and expectations seem to play an important part in sexual performance for both men and women (Hendricks and Hendricks, 1977). A partner's views are particularly important in sustaining a sense of sexual attractiveness.

Satisfactory sex, now defined in terms appropriate for elderly partners rather than the youth-oriented and ageist terms of the early sexologists, is recognized as an important ingredient for late-life satisfaction (Barbara Turner and Catherine Adams, 1983). It has recently been suggested that sexual expression is important for self-esteem, self-acceptance and general wellbeing at all ages, but particularly later on in life when other sources of support might be reduced (Huyck, 1977).

Despite this, we should avoid the risk of overrating sexual activity in old age. The tendency in the course of this century to elevate sexual experience has created new imperatives. In earlier decades, feminist writers referred to 'the tyranny of orgasm' in relation to the demand that women enjoy sexual intercourse in the same way as their partners (Elizabeth Wilson, 1977). The current preoccupation with the quality of sexual experience in old age could be translated into new pressures on older people (Linda Ade-Ridder, 1990; Thienhaus *et al.*, 1986). It might become yet another way of discounting older women for whom, in most cases, sexual activity (apart from masturbation) ceases to be an option on the death of the partner. As we shall see, the options for lesbian women appear to be much wider, since the possibility of finding new partners is not diminished by age.

We know very little about the sexual politics of late-life marriages. Examining power relationships is a new feature which brings the study of elderly couples into line with feminist work on marriage in general. For many older women, a power imbalance has always existed in the marriage. Power plays take different forms, often focusing on an apparently trivial but symbolic item or event. I recently encountered a woman whose husband demanded sole access to the television remote control unit, becoming very angry if she attempted to use it. Their 2-year-old grandson handled it with impunity.

Widowhood

For such women, widowhood may contain an element of relief, although in general the passage from wife to widow is difficult to negotiate. If it happens 'on time', when the majority of the peer group is similarly affected, the strains are less (Zena Blau, 1973; Gloria Heinemann and Patricia Evans, 1990). Widowhood is an expectation for old women in our culture, who still tend to marry men older than themselves despite demographic trends which make this an anachronism (Gibson, 1990). The loss of the partner through death, as through divorce, involves a series of losses: companionship; material support; a partner in a world which is couple-oriented; someone to negotiate on her behalf in a male-dominated society where women often do not acquire the skills necessary to promote their own interests (Jerrome, 1990b). Despite the benefits which marriage confers, most women widowed in late life have no intention of replacing the lost spouse (Helena Lopata, 1980). Their reasons vary from idealization of the former husband to a shortage of suitable men; from fear of conflict between a new partner and adult children, to a reluctance to give up a new-found independence.

At the psychological level, most widows experience pain: of being deserted; of losing a love object; of grief and loneliness. All must deal with the existential problems of bereavement—of finding a meaning in existence and a new identity after the death of a long-term partner (Marris, 1974; Irene Burnside, 1985).

The common response to widowhood is resilience and adaptation. Some women benefit from the help of professionals, but in general a positive outcome and the release of positive potentials in bereavement are a product of the personal resources of the woman and her informal network. For many women, widowhood brings the opportunity to do new things, such as travel. It increases the scope for social participation, particularly with other women.

Friendship and social networks

We expect widows to be lonely. The loss of stable companionship makes them vulnerable. We need to exist in the mind and emotions of others for our mental health, and in western culture it is the long-term partner who is expected to meet that need. Although kin are also important, marriage is the main area of emotional investment in adulthood and is expected to be the main source of emotional fulfilment.

This seems to work in practice, particularly for men. Early studies of confidant relationships revealed interesting gender differences. While married men tended to name their wives as their main source of emotional support, women were as likely to name a friend or an adult child (Jerrome, 1981).

Friendship

Friendship is a major resource for women in later life. There are gender differences in the experience of friendship from childhood onwards. Close friendships between women are characterized by more emotional involvement and self-disclosure: talk is one of the main activities of female friendship (Hess, 1979; Frances Johnson and Elizabeth Aries, 1983). In some ways friendship is even more important for older women than kinship. Kin represent continuity, a sense of identity, and caring which is not contingent on liking or approval. Friends are chosen on the basis of mutual attraction. Their existence is therefore a measure of the worth of the chosen and boosts self-esteem in a way that kin cannot. At points in the life course characterized by change and uncertainty, such as adolescence and the early years of retirement, friends—members of the peer group—play a vital part in managing age-related changes. But friends are important throughout life, their biographies intertwined (M. Jocelyn Armstrong and Karen Goldsteen, 1990; Doris Francis, 1990; Sarah Matthews, 1986). Migration both within and between countries may deprive some older women of this source of life-long friendship.

Friendship is important for older women of all social and cultural backgrounds, although its form and content varies. The special or best friend is both confidante and companion in shared activities: shopping, outings, religious events, scrabble or bridge parties at home, travel and holidays. Often the best-friend relationship is embedded in a network of women friends with shared interests.

The informal network is seen operating in a variety of settings. One is the old people's club, a community of widows. Club-going is a way of life for a minority of retired people, mainly working-class white women. There, the assertiveness which develops over the course of a woman's life (Gutmann, 1987) can be seen in full flower. The members and leaders alike organize their affairs with vigour and a general disregard for the few men present, who are socially invisible. The women benefit from peer-group solidarity, expressed in song, games and dramatic performance (Jerrome, 1988b; 1989). The weekly rituals provide a structure for existence, as well as moral and practical support. An important feature is the chat between friends and over tea. In the course of conversation, personal events are put into perspective.

Club-going is an activity of friendship. Club meetings are attended with friends: the object is less to make new ones than to reinforce existing friendly relations. The expectation conflicts with that of some club leaders whose aim is to integrate lonely people and extend their social networks. In clubs run by charitable organizations such as Age Concern, rival concepts of friendship interfere with the smooth running of the club and the enjoyment of members. For the members, friendship is an exclusive category, expressed through seating patterns ('bagging chairs'). The leaders, on the other hand, aim for an open club in which 'we are all friends together and can sit anywhere'. The members, for whom an open club is a contradiction in terms, make their views felt through such strategies as persistent noise-making and general recalcitrance (Jerrome, 1991).

Concepts of friendship and norms which determine patterns of inclusion and exclusion create difficulties for lonely women who come in search of friendship. Old people's clubs might not be the best source of friends and the truly lonely who have no social connections are rarely to be found there. But ironically those clubs which are set up expressly to create friendships are not necessarily any more successful (Jerrome, 1983; 1991). However, for those older women from minority ethnic groups, who may be isolated by language barriers and/or by the ethnocentricity of most older people's clubs, opportunities to socialize with other women from the same cultural background offer a way to develop new friendships and to counterbalance emotional dependence on kin. Such clubs can provide a safe base where a common language is spoken, religious rituals are observed, familiar food is served and memories can be shared and, most importantly for some, a women-only space.

In general, women's social networks and spheres of influence are inclined to develop as they go through life, if only because the earlier years are characterized by relatively narrow concerns and later years see a removal of some of the constraints on social activities. The end of active parenthood, widowhood and the death of a dependent elderly relative may all release potential for sociability.

There is however some variation in the capacity to make friends. There are women whose friendships continue to multiply. As circumstances change and old relationships lose their significance, new ones are added. Existing ones are maintained in new forms, and social life becomes fuller and richer, offering greater variety and freedom of choice in companionship and areas for emotional investment. Then there are women who, like the first group, are friend-makers. Their relationships have a serial quality: the loss of an old tie as circumstances change is balanced by the acquisition of a new one. The fund of sociability remains roughly the same. The current best friend is dropped and replaced as necessary. The friend-makers tend to be single or widowed women, fit and active, with few family commitments.

There are some women for whom the passage of time involves the gradual attenuation of sociable relationships. Lost friends are not replaced and the source of affection and intimacy gradually diminishes. Women for whom ageing involves a net loss in sociable relationships have certain characteristics. They are socially isolated, either by extreme old age and physical frailty, by an absence of social skills, or by a negative self-image.

Attitudes to ageing, and feelings about themselves as ageing women, seem important in the ability to make friends. Susan Sontag (1978) claimed that the ageing experience is made more difficult for women by the value attached to feminine youth in our culture. On the other hand, the handicap created by the twin processes of ageism and sexism are to some extent balanced by women's emotional strength.

Prevailing attitudes towards femininity clearly do affect a significant number of women whose feelings about themselves isolate them from other women. Unlike the friend-makers, the lonely women share the ageist and sexist values of our society. What matters most to them is being physically attractive in a youthful way and being in service rather than command, both of which are confirmed by the presence of a male attendant (ideally a husband). By these criteria they have failed, as ageing and unattached women, and their lack of self-confidence acts as an additional handicap. The company of other women reminds them of their own inferior status. They have, in any case, never had close women friends, and those acquired to counteract the loneliness of recent years, in a friendship club for instance, share their circumstances. The experience of these women suggests that the usefulness of gender as an explanation for friendship patterns goes beyond the differences between men and women, and accounts for some differences between women themselves.

Loneliness

Acute loneliness is experienced by some older people in situations where we might least expect it: in marriage, in the idyllic retirement home, in the bosom of the multigenerational household (Wenger, 1983). Poverty also limits the capacity for friendship, by reducing the ability to finance the small transactions of social life.

Much has been written about loneliness in old age: its form and pervasiveness, its causes and the possibilities for alleviating it (Jerrome 1990b; 1991). The extent of loneliness in later life tends to be exaggerated, but we know that it is a feature of extreme old age, and is associated with isolation. Some isolated people have always been marginal and the conditions which lie at the root of the problem have accompanied them into old age. 'Shopping bag-women', who store their few possessions in shopping trollies and sleep in shop doorways, are such a group. They appear to see solitariness and the avoidance of both public assistance and personal intimacy as a means of continued control over their own lives, after experiencing intolerable levels of danger and distress in earlier relationships (Jennifer Hand, 1983). Unlike homeless old men, who have more social contacts than is apparent to the casual observer (Blacher, 1983; Cohen, 1989), these homeless women appear to be truly isolated.

Loneliness remains a difficult topic to investigate, although it is recognized as a social problem worthy of study by those who encounter its consequences: depression and stress-related physical illness (Elaine Murphy, 1982; Valerie Grant, 1986). In some ways it appears to be a women's problem. This is not just because there are far more women in the vulnerable categories, but because women appear to have different emotional needs from men. The suggestion is that their self-esteem requires acceptance and approval by others to a greater extent than is the case with men, and that they therefore invest more heavily in relationships. The work of feminist psychotherapists relates this to early experience in identity formation. The absence of clear boundaries between mothers and daughters can result in unsatisfied cravings for intimacy which persist throughout life and are transmitted from generation to generation (Nancy Chodorow, 1978; Louise Eichenbaum and Susie Orbach, 1985). We have yet to use these ideas to illuminate loneliness in elderly women.

Older lesbian women

The search for intimacy has led some other women in a different direction. The lives of older lesbians, affected as they have been by shifts in popular and official attitudes towards homosexuality, have received little attention in the UK. However it seems from recent biographical writings (Hall Carpenter Archives Lesbian Oral History Group, 1989; Suzanne Nield and Rosalind Pearson, 1992) that the American findings drawn upon in this section may be mirrored here. Although we use the term 'lesbian' it is important to recognize that some older women might prefer to be described as 'gay'. 'Lesbian' was a stigmatized word in their youth. It became more widely used but also acquired political overtones in the 1960s and 1970s.

Identity

Earlier this century sex was seldom talked about and girls knew very little about expressing their sexuality except through marriage (Buffy

Dunker, 1987). Even those who felt 'different' tended to marry, for a host of reasons: to avoid the hazards of experimental sex and premarital pregnancy; or of becoming an old maid; or wondering if they were lesbian. The word itself had negative connotations and was generally not used. Sharley McLean, born in 1923, thought lesbian 'was some sort of swear word' (Hall Carpenter Archives Lesbian Oral History Group, 1989). In the 1930s the term lesbian suggested decadence, inversion and vice. McLean and her friends were aware of their attraction for each other but had no name for their feelings or identity. The established middle-aged couples they heard referred to as 'homosexual ladies' had nothing to do with 'us girls'. For some young women, Radclyffe Hall's 'The Well of Loneliness' was a formative influence. Recognizing themselves in the characters was a powerful emotional experience, although popular responses to the book did not encourage self-disclosure.

There is much in the autobiographical accounts of early lesbian lives which confirms the impression of danger in the pursuit of intimacy. The dangers involved in 'coming out' persuaded most lesbians to remain 'in the closet'. The absence of a visible network and subculture created enormous difficulties for those who actively sought new women friends like themselves. One response was to gravitate towards certain occupations which were thought attractive to lesbians, such as the armed forces.

In the 1940s and 1950s, in the UK as well as in the USA, lesbians who were 'out' organized their lives in terms of the dominant heterosexual model, with its division of labour along masculine and feminine lines. In the decade of the 1950s this role-playing was an important part of lesbian culture. The division into butch and femme, with gender-specific dress and mannerisms, provided an identifiable grouping and was a source of strength and pride. It alienated some would-be joiners, particularly those whose preferences did not match the butch–femme stereotypes. In the absence of alternative lifestyles, women who did not fit in did not identify themselves as lesbian (Nield and Pearson, 1992).

In the 1960s, the emergence of the gay bars symbolizing independence provided a communal life style and models for behaviour which had been lacking in earlier decades. Attracting both men and women, the bars could be found in Paris and Berlin, in London and in Brighton, as well as in San Francisco, Chicago and other big cities. The culture of these bars has since been cited as an important stage in the emergence of a lesbian identity (Joan Nestle, 1988). Valuable support of a different kind was also beginning to develop in the form of clubs, pressure groups and lesbian publications. The Daughters of Bilitis in the USA, and the broadsheet Arena III in England helped women to assert themselves in a new way (Hall Carpenter Archives Lesbian Oral History Group, 1989).

The Gay Liberation Movement, the Women's Movement and the growing social acceptance of homosexuality throughout the 1960s and 1970s made it possible to live more openly as a lesbian. Many of today's older lesbians came out in these decades. They talk of the immense relief on shedding the burden of deceit and hypocrisy. There was a new freedom to experiment with new roles in the couple relationship. This was experienced as a unique opportunity to be themselves. But these were dangerous times, too. A response to coming out at work, for example, was often dismissal by hitherto progressive employers (Bob Cant and Susan Hemmings, 1988).

These women report few regrets about not coming out for so long, despite the loneliness and frustration of their earlier years. Indeed, the current generation of aged lesbians have often been married, but the costs of the double life they had to lead are to some extent counterbalanced by the existence of children and grandchildren. For some, the choice to marry was deliberate:

'I have no sadness that it wasn't easier to be gay when I was young. I really wanted to have children. But I think for the women who didn't take my path, the women who really wanted to live with other women and be with them, it was very hard . . .' (Mary Flick in Marcy Adelman, 1986, p.23).

Despite the advances of the 1970s and 1980s, coming out has never been easy in a heterosexist and patriarchal culture. The emerging lesbian is beset by silence, lies, isolation, intimidation and physical violence, while self-doubt assails her from within. Older lesbian women talk of the shock of falling in love with another woman, after 'drifting along with the social current for thirty years', and of the problem of telling other loved ones such as daughters (Nield and Pearson, 1992). There was relief when they seemed to know already and did not reject their mothers, and sadness when they did.

Ageing lesbians have, over the decades, experienced enormous discontinuity in their public personae. The resurgent homophobia, related to mass hysteria about public health and HIV/AIDS and expressed in provisions such as Section 28, creates new risks. There is a sense of being pushed back into the bleak early days of 'lies, secrets, silence' (Hall Carpenter Archives Lesbian Oral History Group, 1989) and it might still be preferable for the older lesbian who is still in the closet to stay where she is: her choice should be respected.

Relationships

Although lesbianism tends today to be defined exclusively in terms of sexual attraction, there is considerable variation in the degree of sexual involvement in lesbian relationships. Seen very much as romantic friendship in the eighteenth and nineteenth centuries, when other women were possibly the only source of 'pure, unmixed tenderness', lesbianism is still perhaps best characterized by the element of romantic love (Uncovering Lesbian History Publications Group, 1986).

Some women discover lesbianism in midlife. Middle-aged married women may define themselves as lesbian without any homosexual experience (Martha Kirkpatrick, 1989). Their desires, recognized, emerge powerfully in midlife to prompt the active search for a female partner. Sometimes a life-threatening or disfiguring illness such as breast cancer has been the trigger for deciding that the quality of intimacy and support in an existing marriage is not good enough. Sometimes the wish for closeness with another woman has always been there but suppressed until children were mature enough to understand or leave behind. In some cases a chance meeting with another bisexual woman has awakened dormant feelings. They establish lesbian relationships despite the possible loss of the heterosexual support system and the disbelief and disapproval of family and friends.

Yet the woman who adopts a lesbian lifestyle in middle age often becomes part of a network of lesbian friends who provide support and companionship. As we have seen, the existence of friends in retirement is life-preserving for all women. Their presence may be more important for morale than that of adult children and other kin. For elderly lesbians this is doubly so, since friends may act as substitute kin, as well as providing a shared identity and a supportive ideology. Most women in Sharon Raphael and Mina Robinson's study (1984) reported weak sibling ties and strong friendship ties (although ties with children also remained strong), and it is those women who had the highest self-esteem.

According to the popular stereotype, the quality of life in lesbian old age is poor: loneliness and isolation lie ahead of the woman whose adult years are spent loving other women, lacking in the comforts of a 'normal' home life, lacking children. The truth can be very different. The onset of old age may find them, like many other older women, independent and resourceful, although sometimes anxious about continuing financial support in deep old age. They tend to be more involved in leisure-time activities and thus connected to more sources of personal satisfaction (Sagir and Robins, 1973).

Meeting other women and recognizing them as kindred spirits is one of the greatest difficulties the older lesbian faces. Recognition of potential partners was particularly difficult in earlier decades when the need for secrecy limited the possibilities. The problem was partly practical: how could women meet in suitable circumstances when they were passing as heterosexual, with the full range of commitments of marriage and family life? The workplace—particularly in female-dominated occupations such as nursing, social work and some service and manufacturing industries—was and still is an important source of lesbian friends and lovers. More than half of the lesbians in Beth Schneider's study (1984) had had at least one sexual relationship with a person from work. The absence of a workplace in the lives of retired lesbians is a factor to be borne in mind when considering the social needs of older women.

Sexual satisfaction continues to be important for some older lesbians, who enjoy an increasing pool of potential partners (Raphael and Robinson, 1984). Although physical changes cause the kinds of concerns common to all ageing women, there appears to be a greater degree of mutual acceptance within the elderly peer group. For some younger lesbians too, age enhances attractiveness: the grey haired woman has mystique and is an object of desire.

The couple relationship

Contrary to popular belief, most older lesbians are coupled. Indeed some older lesbians will have been with their current partners for thirty years or more. The typical pattern is to have moved through several partnerships, lasting between a couple of years and some decades. However, while women in heterosexual partnerships are apt to complain of loneliness and a lack of communication, lesbian couples can suffer from the opposite: excessive intensity and a lack of privacy (Barbara Sang, 1984; Kirkpatrick, 1989). There may be a tendency to merge psychologically with the partner, leading to a loss of the sense of separateness and an inability to express or tolerate differences. It seems ironic that the quality of closeness sought in the heterosexual marriage and admired as an expression of true love can be damaging in women who love each other. The idealization of merger in the romantic ideal, with its loss of boundaries between self and partner, may restrict women's growth. In many lesbian relationships similarities are overvalued and differences diminished and often feared. Despite an ideology of independence and selfhood the struggle towards autonomy may be full of conflict (Kirkpatrick, 1989).

Such relationship problems are not exclusive to lesbians. Non-sexual friendships between women tend also to demand conformity, but to a lesser extent. Women are supposed to care for others, and they are constantly concerned with the question of whether they are giving enough. As a result of this it takes more strength in female relationships to take care of one's own needs and not always be there for the other. The romantic ideal of self-sacrifice contributes to a powerful dynamic in a relationship that all women need to recognize.

In the same way that an individual woman may hesitate to come out, so also older lesbian couples may be under pressure to remain invisible. Lesbian relationships are not legally recognized: a fact which leads to much discrimination against, and difficulties for, older lesbian women. For example, the terminal illness of a long-term partner may not be acknowledged as creating the same stresses for her friend as it might in a heterosexual couple, and access to the bedside might need to be fought for. Visiting rules which specify only the immediate family may make it difficult for lesbian partners to continue caring at the point when it is most important. Practical arrangements may be taken over by relatives who know far less than her partner about the wishes of the dying woman. From the funeral itself to the disposal of personal belongings and sale of the property, the interests of the bereaved partner often are not only ignored but are without legal status.

Autobiographical accounts by aged lesbians are full of poignancy. But strength and sturdiness are also features of their lives. The women witness the physical decline and death of friends and lovers with a sense of aloneness that comes from being both old and lesbian. In the words of Barbara MacDonald, 'I never grew old before; never died before. I don't really know how it's done' (MacDonald and Rich, 1984, p.19). When these women were young, their lesbian elders were dispersed and invisible. Now they are old themselves and their 'Great to be Gray' badges, worn with pride at gay rallies, demand recognition and respect.

Conclusion

The demographic changes which have produced an ageing society have their cultural counterpart. Our attention has been drawn to the impact of change on what it means to be old (Featherstone and Hepworth, 1989; Bernice Martin, 1990). We have seen how the contemporary life course calls for a deconstruction of some of our accepted categories, such as grandmother. Just as the concept of old age has acquired new meanings in the latter part of the twentieth century, so we might expect relationships in later life to shift in significance. Since larger numbers of women enter retirement in the company of their peers, we might expect the age-segregation which is a feature of our society to be reflected in intensified peer-group activity. This suggests at least one new key dyad, that of friendship between women, in addition to the accepted ones of husband–wife and mother–daughter. Some would identify yet another, the tie between siblings.

The flexibility demanded in our thinking about social arrangements in late twentieth century society extends to other areas of experience. The rigidity of our sexual categories—homosexual and heterosexual —drew comment several decades ago. Writers like Pat Caplan (1987) refer to the fluidity of sexual identities in earlier times and other cultures and note the failure of our own society to cope with sexual ambiguity, thus forcing individuals to identify themselves in terms of simple dichotomies. Lesbianism has been presented as both a sexual orientation and a special kind of friendship. If we view it as one kind of sociable relationship between women, on a continuum between sexual and non-sexual friendship, we see that the similarities between older women are greater than their differences.

6 Caring: a legitimate interest of older women

Gillian Dalley

'. . . I retired on January 28th. I was sixty-four years and six months, not exactly 65. And I went to India. When I came back my husband was very seriously ill. So for eight years I worked for my husband, I didn't do anything else . . . Yes it was very hard work . . . Because you can't satisfy a patient. Whatever you do, the patient always thinks that it's not enough. I did not regret it . . . Sometimes I became a little upset, when he wasn't happy. Otherwise no. Because he was altogether a changed person. When he became sick he was not the same man he used to be . . . He was a very, very brave man . . .'

(Charanjit)

Introduction

Women have a very real and legitimate interest in the whole issue of caring. First, there is an ideology of caring which has underpinned many of the social forms of care which prevail today: it is one which favours women's leading role and the pre-eminence of family-based models of care. Second, there is enough persuasive evidence to show that women have and still do bear the greater burden of providing care although clearly men have a part to play. Third, there is evidence that women themselves are the largest recipients of care once they reach old age. Thus, at certain stages of their lives women provide care, often at considerable cost to themselves and, at a later stage, they are the people often in most need of care.

There are many mixed demands being made upon women, both now and in coming years: one arm of official policy supports the idea of drawing women into the labour force more and more, while another stresses the importance of informal care. This presupposes that there will be a plentiful supply of home-based, non-working people (women) available to be informal carers for the growing numbers of frail elderly people. It is the impact on women of current government policy relating to community care (both formal and informal) that is the focus of this chapter. We critically examine the origins of community-care policies before analysing the particular contribution of women to informal caring. The caring relationship is explored both from the perspective of the carers and the recipients of care. The chapter concludes with a discussion of the tensions between collective and individualistic approaches to the social care needs of frail older people.

The origins of community-care policies

Although the origin of community-care policies can be traced back to the early 1960s and before, the impact that they would have on women was not recognized until the late 1970s. It is generally agreed that changes in the treatment of mental illness, with the introduction of new drug therapies and the insights of a number of psychiatrists leading to the view that mentally ill people did not have to be kept in locked wards (Kathleen Jones, 1972), marked the start of community care. This was built into official government policy in 1962 (Ministry of Health, 1962) when Enoch Powell, health minister at the time, announced a fifteen-year programme of hospital bed closures, with the expectation that patients would in future be cared for within the community. The policy of maintaining or returning people to be cared for in the community became accepted by practitioners and policy-makers alike.

The policy became even more appealing during the 1970s with the growing recognition that the numbers of people requiring care would grow in following years, partly in the belief that community care would be cheaper than costly hospital provision. Successive governments published white papers advocating the policy for people who, in the terminology of the time, were described as having a 'mental handicap' (DHSS, 1971), mental illness (DHSS, 1975) and who were elderly (DHSS, 1978). In addition, in a significant policy development in 1976, the Labour government set as a major goal for the health and personal social services a strategy which planned to give priority to what had become known as the 'Cinderella' services—those which cared for elderly, mentally ill, and disabled people and those with learning difficulties (DHSS, 1976).

At the outset, community care was seen as a process of reducing the number of hospital places devoted to the care of these client groups. The policy was elaborated over time and took on a more positive aspect. A set of rights and expectations came to be associated with it. The 1976 white paper for example, set out the form of care it believed people with learning difficulties had the right to expect. It listed fifteen principles on which it believed policy should be based, and included the belief that each person 'should live with his own family as long as this does not impose an undue burden on them or him'.

Practitioners in the fields of learning difficulties, mental illness and the care of elderly people supported the ideas associated with the policies. The Jay Report, in 1979, relying extensively on the views of experts in the field, put forward what it referred to as an 'unashamedly idealistic' model of care; likewise, the white paper 'A Happier Old Age', published in 1978, stressed the value of maintaining elderly people in the community.

A key concept, developed by Michael Bayley (1973), was the distinction that could be made between care in the community and care by the community. It was the latter that underlay much of the thinking about community care that developed during this period. The series of documents published by the Conservative government after 1979 accepted its significance explicitly. Growing Older (DHSS, 1981), for example, stated:

> 'The primary sources of support and care for elderly people are informal and voluntary. These spring from the personal ties of kinship, friendship and neighbourhood . . . Care in the community must increasingly mean care by the community' (p.3).

Official policy, then, was beginning to recognize the significance of the role to be played by the informal sector. It was beginning to recognize the role of carers, and it also recognized that most of them were women:

> 'When help is needed, families are, as they have always been, the principal source of support and care . . . It may often involve considerable personal sacrifice, particularly where the "family" is one person, often a single woman, caring for an elderly relative' (DHSS, 1981, p.37).

The 1980s witnessed yet more policy reports, together with a growing critique of community care. In particular the Audit Commission (1986) identified a number of formidable barriers to the development of community care, arguing that radical change was needed and suggesting that possible strategies should be independently examined (Melanie Henwood, 1990a). During this decade too, more research evidence was being amassed which continued to highlight the inadequacies of institutional care (Godlove et al., 1982; Booth, 1985). This also helped fuel the drive towards recent community-care policies and legislation (Griffiths, 1988; Department of Health, 1988; NHS and Community Care Act, 1990). However, whether the continuing rhetoric of support for informal carers can be translated into reality remains to be seen.

The recognition of informal care

At the beginning of the 1980s, carers became fashionable. Before then their presence was assumed but barely noticed. While care in the community was now widely advocated, 'the community' had not been scrutinized in any detail: who within 'the community' did the caring was not often made explicit. But by the end of the 1970s, things began to change: public attention came to be focused on the needs of elderly and disabled people and the people who cared for them. Suddenly the issue of caring became the centre of much social policy debate. Perhaps it was partly because government policy had finally come round to addressing the issue, but it was also due to the fact that feminists and others interested in women's rights had already become concerned. Up till that time, most feminists had concentrated on the role of women in the domestic sphere as carers of children and servicers of menfolk, and the relation of these roles to women's place in the labour market (Elizabeth Wilson, 1977).

One of the first signs of interest in other aspects of women's caring role was a paper by Janet Finch and Dulcie Groves (1980) suggesting that community-care policies militated against equal opportunities between the sexes because they relied on women's unpaid domestic labour. The Equal Opportunities Commission (EOC) also began to be concerned about the issue around the same time, publishing a survey report of a sample of people 'caring for elderly and handicapped dependants' (EOC, 1980). It pointed out that up until that time most studies had focused upon the problems and needs of those client groups requiring care. This study was different it stated, because it concentrated on the needs and problems of those providing the care, saying 'most of the carers are, of course, women'. The EOC published two further reports furnishing more details of the reality of informal caring and setting out a series of recommendations for support services that ought to be available to carers (EOC, 1982a; 1982b).

These were closely followed by a number of studies looking at the conceptual aspects of caring: Hilary Graham (1983) examined the psychological forces which encourage women into the caring role and Clare Ungerson (1983) looked at the ideological and political influences which lead women to feel responsibility for caring. Hilary Land and Hilary Rose (1985) discussed what they called the 'compulsory altruism' that impels women to take on caring responsibilities in a society which is founded at every level on an expectation of women's willingness to deny themselves for the sake of others. The essence of their feminist view is that there are many unspoken assumptions underlying society's approach to caring which place a disproportionate burden of responsibility upon women. Traditional roles and expectations have tended to place women in the domestic sphere, where they have been concerned with caring and servicing tasks. Similar tasks in the public sphere have then become women's responsibility by extension; hence the predominantly female labour force to be found at the lower levels of the health and social services.

The pervading ideology is thus one which sees caring as primarily a domestic task (and thus a gendered task); this then fuels more generalized attitudes towards informal caring. The 'family-based model of care' (Gillian Dalley, 1988) has become the only model of value. Other forms, such as institutional or group forms of care, have been rendered unacceptable, partly because they have failed in terms of their own standards but also because they do not meet ideological norms either. Community care, as we have described earlier, is founded on this general principle. 'Dependent' people are best cared for in their own homes, preferably by members of their own families. Failing this, surrogate family forms are deemed to be appropriate. Hostels and group homes are only made acceptable by being modelled on family forms; elderly people are said to live in 'family-like' surroundings in geriatric wards that have been made 'homely' with carpets and divan beds. Varied forms of care are rendered suitable by being cast in the mould of the family-based model.

Feminists and others argue that there is nothing wrong with informal caring located in the home and performed by close relatives, be they women or men, as long as they do it willingly, free from pressure and the feeling of moral obligation. As the EOC said in relation to women in particular, 'it does not suggest that women give up caring; it does suggest that the responsibility for care should be shared more equally, and that those who willingly take up this responsibility should be adequately supported and protected' (EOC, 1982b, p.1). However, they would also argue for a more sympathetic and positive view being taken of other forms of care, both as a means of resolving the problems associated with informal caring and also because other forms of care might offer choice and variety to those needing care. This will be taken up in a later section.

Who cares and who is cared for?

Demographic forces mean that during the present decade and beyond, the numbers of elderly people, especially those who are very elderly, will increase proportionate to the rest of the population. In association with this, the number of younger people coming into the labour force will decline. Many very elderly people will require considerable support of both the medico-nursing and social kind, and there is an expectation that women, the only 'spare capacity' in the system at the moment, will provide this. And yet there are contradictions in these expectations—and major implications for women who have to come to terms with them.

Caring is generally considered a women's issue and it can be argued that it is predominantly an older women's issue. More women than men are carers and more women (mostly elderly) than men are cared for; this is likely to be the case for the foreseeable future. However the data available on who cares and is cared for are complex to analyse. When interest in the issue of caring first developed it was widely stated, with little qualification, that it was predominantly a women's issue because women constituted the substantial majority of carers. Yet studies that were carried out at the time did not demonstrate conclusively that women did form the substantial majority of carers. It has to be said however that these surveys tended to be small in scale and not necessarily representative of the wider caring/cared-for population.

The 1980 EOC study, for example (based on a 36 per cent response to a randomly selected sample of 2500 households in West Yorkshire) found that 141 households contained a carer. Of the 116 carers interviewed three-quarters were found to be women and one-quarter men. Twenty-seven daughters looked after elderly parents compared with six sons. Children constituted 12 per cent of the care recipients and all were looked after by their mothers, with the equal help, in one case, of a father.

A subsequent EOC study compared the experiences of a sample of men and women carers identified from a sample of 255 elderly people already in contact with the services and therefore not randomly selected. The split between male and female carers was much less marked in this study: 59 per cent were women as opposed to 41 per cent men (Ann Charlesworth *et al.*, 1984).

Other frequently cited studies were not concerned to distinguish between male and female carers. Jane Lewis and Barbara Meredith (1988) interviewed 41 women who had cared for their mothers; Cherrill Hicks (1988) surveyed more than 80 carers (of both genders) drawn through personal contacts of various sorts. These studies were more concerned to explore the experience (particularly the burdens) of caring rather than draw conclusions about hard figures.

It has been the data derived from the 1985 GHS (OPCS, 1987a) of informal carers that have provided the most often quoted figures. Hazel Green's analysis (1988) shows that there are about six million carers in the UK, with 1.7 million caring for someone in the same household. More particularly it found substantial numbers of men who reported they were carers—12 per cent of men compared with 15 per cent of women. Absolute numbers of women carers are greater (3.5 million women compared with 2.5 million men) because of the larger proportion of women in the general population. The evidence then, seems incontrovertible; the arguments of feminists and others, that caring is predominantly a women's issue seem superficially at least, to be less than secure.

But the GHS data bear further scrutiny. The broad figures above include all care recipients, be they adults or children, and relate to care in its broadest aspects; from heavy personal care (washing, lifting, feeding), to keeping an eye on the frail person, as well as looking after paperwork or financial matters and keeping company. In respect of the more arduous aspects of caring, for example, women do appear to take greater responsibility for personal care (20 per cent more female than male carers). In addition, in the peak age group for caring (45–64 years), significantly more women than men were carers (24 per cent compared with 16 per cent), with more of them providing care for at least 20 hours a week. Substantially more single women than single men in this age group (29 per cent compared with 16 per cent) were also carers. Furthermore, sole carers who are women (60 per cent of women compared with 46 per cent of men) were shown to be less financially well off than their male equivalents.

Maria Evandrou (1990) has suggested, citing Gillian Parker of York University, that there may be flaws in the way the GHS data have been collected in the first place. According to this argument, the screening question is phrased 'rather liberally': it asks about people who 'look after or give special help to' or 'provide some regular service or help for any sick, handicapped person', adult or child. Evandrou (and Parker) suggest that women and men may respond differently to such a question. Women see the caring that they do as part of their 'normal' duties whereas men regard it as something extra, which they would therefore be more likely to report.

Although the GHS survey broke down the caring tasks into various categories, there was not enough published detail as to the relation between the gender and age of the carer, the type of help given and the number of hours per week devoted to it. Some recent secondary analysis, however, has shed light on these issues (Sara Arber and Jay Ginn, 1991a; Janet Askham *et al.*, 1992). First, this indicates that 12 per cent of women and 9 per cent of men provide informal care to people over the age of 65. While confirming the major role of women aged between 45–64 years (28 per cent of carers), Arber and Ginn emphasize the significant contributions of both older women and men to informal care. They show that people over the age of 65 provide 35 per cent of the informal care needed by other elderly people. Amongst this age group the gender differences are less marked, with 19 per cent of older women and 16 per cent of older men providing care. The main factor accounting for this is spouse care, which is undertaken almost equally by older women and men. Second, Arber and Ginn draw attention to the differences in the care provided. Eighty per cent of informal carers support an elderly person in a separate household and provide on average 9 hours care per week compared with the average 53 hours spent by a carer in the same household. There is a negligible gender difference in the time spent by spouses, but in other relationships both within and between households there is a consistent gender difference, with women of all ages providing considerably more care. However, there are insufficient data to differentiate between the caring tasks that are the response to disability and what may be seen as part of the ordinary give and take of family support. Arber and Ginn's analysis cautions against popular conceptions of older people both as a 'burden' on society and as non-contributing, highly dependent recipients of informal care.

We also need to consider the degree to which the 'cared for' older population is gender-differentiated. For example, 42 per cent of carers were looking after women over the age of 75, whereas only 12 per cent were looking after men in this age group. This demonstrates the greater longevity of women over men; it also explains the relatively large proportion of men caring for elderly women rather than the reverse. More men have elderly wives to care for than wives have elderly husbands to care for because men die earlier.

A further difficulty with the available information is the lack of detail provided about black and minority ethnic communities in relation to the numbers of elderly people who are, or are likely to be, in need of care, and the numbers of informal carers (both female and male) already providing care. Yet again, as in so many other areas of social policy, people from the black and minority ethnic communities and their needs remain hidden (Alison Norman, 1985; Cherrill Hicks, 1988). Two small-scale studies in Leicester (Bould, 1990) and in Southwark (Joy Ann McCalman, 1990) indicate similar caring patterns of and by women while emphasizing that traditional obligations may place greater social pressure on minority ethnic women than on their white sisters. Joy Ann McCalman interviewed 35 carers from within the Afro-Caribbean, Asian and Chinese/Vietnamese communities. Approximately 62 per cent were women and a similar percentage were over 40 years of age. All the elderly people were related to the carer and 77 per cent lived within the same household. The majority of carers spent over 11 hours per day caring for their relative. There is strong evidence both in this study and in Bould's against the prevailing norm that extended family networks make caring easier. Most carers rarely had a break and received little practical support from other family members.

For a policy based on the presumed availability of informal carers, there is another major issue to take into account. Many elderly people do not have relatives to care for them, and as they get older the more this becomes evident. For example, Mark Abrams (1978) found that 30 per cent of elderly people in his sample had never had children or had no living children. Isobel Allen and her colleagues (1992) found that 22 per cent of their sample who were living in the community, and a third of those living in residential homes, either had never borne children or had no living children. Reliance on informal care from close relatives was surprisingly infrequent. Forty per cent of those who said they had close relatives reported that they received no help from them—and it should be noted that the sample of those living in the community consisted of elderly people regarded as being on the margins of requiring residential care. In these circumstances, elderly women are especially vulnerable because of their greater longevity.

From the perspective of the individual woman, the sense of involvement in a continuing cycle of caring (as provider and recipient) is overwhelming. In spite of women's increased and increasing participation in the labour market, they still hold predominant responsibility for child-rearing. A woman's responsibilities in relation to children may also not be complete when her own children have grown up; in middle age she may find she has responsibilities, as grandmother to a new generation of children (see pp.88–91). At the same time, she may also be entering a period when she finds she has new caring responsibilities in the opposite direction—towards her parents or other older relatives. She is a woman 'in the middle' in Elaine Brody's terms (1981), a woman of middle age, middle generation, between children and her own parents, who is subject to the competing demands of children (and their children), ageing parents and her own need to work.

As women grow older, they often have to continue with their caring responsibilities. For example, Fay Wright (1986) interviewed a 75-year-old woman who was still caring for her mother, by then almost 100 years old. They may also become infirm themselves and thus the cycle proceeds. Their own daughters (or sons) may begin to care for them; those whose spouses survive may care for them, or they may have to care for their spouses. Or they may survive to live alone and unsupported, or reliant on the limited care offered by friends and neighbours. We know that the number of very elderly women living alone without near relatives is large (see p.87). They have no close relatives to fulfil what might be called 'family obligations' (Finch, 1989) to care for them.

This is likely to mean that the impact of caring may be considerable, especially since women tend to take on the more arduous aspects of caring (personal care, for example) and are more likely to be sole carers. There is limited quantitative evidence about how far women tailor their work around their caring duties in middle age, the extent to which they give up employment in order to care, or its impact in later life. Thus it is hard to judge the full extent of the costs (both psychological and financial) of caring. Some qualitative studies, as well as providing vivid evidence of the emotional costs involved, do look at the issue of employment: Fay Wright's study of female carers (1986) found that one-third of those below retirement age had found it necessary to give up work. It depicts lives deprived of social contact, loss of ambition and impoverishment (Caroline Glendinning, 1992).

The caring relationship

The caring relationship is just that—a relationship. And relationships are made up of feelings and attitudes. In some, the balance of power may be unequal, to the disadvantage of the weaker partner. In others, the dependency of one may be offset by the strength of the other, so that both are complementary. Emotions may be mixed, changeable and often heightened. The circumstances of particular relationships will condition how they are played out. It is important to remember the complexity and variation found in the caring relationship. It is easy to generalize about the 'burden of caring' on the one hand or the 'wish for independence' on the other; there may be a tendency to see caring relationships through a rosy filter just as much as there may be an inclination to see them as minefields of unrelieved gloom.

It is helpful, therefore, to try and disentangle some of these preconceptions. The emotional dimension of caring will depend on many factors: the kinship relationship (father, mother, daughter, son, siblings, spouses and so on); the ages of those involved (parent caring for grown up son or daughter, daughter or son caring for elderly parents, elderly spouse caring for elderly spouse); the particular physical or mental condition of the person being cared for; the degree of outside help available (respite care, other family members, neighbours, day care, domiciliary care); the psychological history of the earlier relationship (dislike, love, hatred, affection); gender (daughter caring for father, son caring for mother, daughter caring for mother, mother caring for daughter, father caring for daughter, parents caring for son and so on); and personal predilection (wanting to be cared for, wanting to be independent, unwilling to care, guilt about unwillingness to care, sense of obligation, resentment at being cared for, acquiescence).

The blend of these particular circumstances and attitudes and how they change over time will determine the exact nature of the caring relationship. Not every relationship will be characterized by one person's guilt or resentment and the other person's unreasonable expectations or high level of dependency. Not every relationship will be suffused with mutual love and support, and a sense of interdependence. Where there is mutual acceptance of the particular circumstances involved, then there may be no problem. Problems arise when there is asymmetry in a relationship, and one partner feels frustrated or overwhelmed by involvement in that relationship.

One of the difficulties for people in caring relationships is that they may harbour many mixed and conflicting feelings at one and the same time. Love may be mixed with feelings of obligation; dislike may be mixed with duty; exhaustion may overwhelm friendship. Many people have written movingly about the stresses placed on relationships by the responsibilities of caring and being cared for.

In the study by Isobel Allen and her colleagues (1992), they report the views of some of the elderly women interviewed about their experiences of being cared for by their informal carers. They resented their dependence on relatives to whom they did not feel particularly close:

> 'I have a cousin—we've never been close . . . He doesn't come often . . . Once I lost my pension book. Now he keeps it and sends me money. It annoys me—he's bossy. I like to be independent' (p.15).

In other cases they expressed their frustration at the way they were regarded by others. One elderly woman described how she felt about losing control over her own life:

> 'When you get old you don't know about these things. Maybe I could have told you once, but I forget things now. When you get old, people don't think of you as a whole person the same as them' (p.47).

The general picture emerging from the study is one of elderly people having little opportunity to make decisions for themselves about their futures and very little choice indeed about what options might be open to them.

For those receiving care, there are pressures—not often, however, recorded in the literature, particularly in the case of elderly people. Younger disabled people have recently been developing a louder voice, graphically describing their experience of informal care. Given the opportunity, older people might make similar observations. Ann Shearer (1982) for example, quotes the words of Bernard Brett:

> 'There are few less pleasant things than to be cared for by somebody who is constantly tired and under too much strain. This makes life tense, unpleasant and unfulfilled' (p.44).

Nasa Begum (1991), a young disabled woman, presents the experiences of other women in similar circumstances. A mother, for example, describes how difficult it is to reconcile herself to the fact that her son has to attend to her needs:

'Although I love my son dearly I feel very guilty that I need him to do such personal things for me. It changes the whole relationship between mother and son' (p.5).

Nasa Begum quotes another young woman, describing how her relationship with her care-providing parents inhibits her own adult development:

'Recent absence of family care has made me feel better about myself as an adult. With family comments I found it impossible to even contemplate sexually based relationships. It makes me feel ashamed and guilty when some aspects of my health are commented on' (p.9).

Not all caring relationships however are restrictive, antagonistic or one-sided. There is some evidence of what Hazel Qureshi and Alan Walker (1989) describe as 'bonds of reciprocity, affection and trust' (p.146) that counters the notion that elderly care-recipients inevitably feel dependent and a burden on those who provide care. In particular, Qureshi and Walker found that where elderly people described their families as 'close' this tended to be associated with receiving assistance. Reciprocity though was one of the main bases of the caring relationship, with past assistance given by the elderly person often being related to current help from carers.

Some carers of elderly people also feel very positive about the quality of the relationship they have with the person they care for. In Qureshi and Walker's study (1989) one daughter describes the emotional closeness she feels for her father in these terms:

'My relationship with my father has never changed since I were born. We've just been good friends all our life kind of thing, you know. It's no use me telling you it changes because it doesn't' (p.155).

Other carers who are not blood relatives also experience emotionally close relationships; for example, the daughter-in-law here talking about her in-laws:

'When they've talked to anybody else about us, they, well me and my sister-in-law, they've talked of us more as daughters than daughters-in-law. They've always said we've taken the place of daughters that they didn't have, you see' (Qureshi and Walker, 1989, p.157).

Nevertheless, many people feel the pressures of being care-providers in caring relationships. In part it is the result of the lack of external support, but also it is the result of the dynamics of the actual relationships in which they are involved. The feelings described here are precisely the mirror image of the feelings expressed by many care-recipients involved in similar caring relationships.

Patricia Slack (Slack and Mulville, 1988), for example, describes how for six years after her mother had suffered a stroke at the age of 75 she had to juggle the responsibilities of caring, arranging outside care to come in, housekeeping, maintaining her relationship with her husband and keeping her job going. Although she loved her mother dearly, enjoyed her company and never doubted her own resolve to provide care, she nevertheless recognized the burden it placed on her as an individual:

> 'I felt tired and longed for some time to myself . . . I needed new under-wear and I had not bought a new item of clothing for three years—there was no time for me to browse along in the shops. My hair had grown long because I had not time or money for hairdressers—I bundled it up with pins and clips and left it to its own devices. I avoided looking in the mirror. In 1980 I was a self-confident young and lively woman; now; three years later, my confidence had ebbed and I was grey and middle-aged. I noticed my memory had deteriorated' (p.136).

In her study of people caring for relatives at home, Cherrill Hicks (1988) quotes extensively from a wide variety of different sorts of caring circumstances—parents caring for children, daughters for mothers, husbands looking after wives and so on. Talking about looking after her mother, a single woman aged 47 described how their relationship had intensified as her mother grew more dependent:

> 'We're very alike, we talk a lot, that's one of the problems—it's very much like a marriage. The sort of relationship I was living before was a normal, independent adult life, even though we were in the same house. The emotional relationship was not so intense. I'm worried about whether I'll be able to cope when she dies' (p.57).

In another case, a 39-year-old man described the role reversal which had taken place since he had taken over care of his elderly mother suffering from Alzheimer's disease. It broke the normal cultural taboos on both gender and generational distance which was hard to take for both of them:

> 'At the beginning it was very difficult: can you imagine having to wipe your own mother's backside, clean her, change her? . . . It was a gradual process. Now she's become like a wee wain' (p.164).

Caring for confused elderly people whose health gradually deterio-rates over years demands significant emotional adjustments as well as increased practical support. Enid Levin and her colleagues (1989) found that the majority of carers were distressed about the situation arising from their relative's illness. One daughter explained that what upset her most was: 'The lack of communication—when we speak we don't seem to touch' (p.51).

Nevertheless, most carers got some satisfaction from the support they gave. The most common reward was the comfort and contentment of their relatives. As one son described it:

'The odd occasion when she does realize you're doing things for her she'll just say, for instance, Oh, you're ever so kind. That's very satisfying. And she always seems ever so pleased to see you when she comes home from day care' (p.52).

There is another aspect. Cherrill Hicks (1988) also describes the isolation that many people from minority ethnic groups feel when they are caring for relatives, especially if they speak little English and have little contact with any support services. Even where services are available, it may be hard for people to take advantage of them. Bharti Hiram, a Hindu woman caring for her 80-year-old mother-in-law pointed out that although there was a day centre that her mother-in-law could go to, she was too frightened to go because she did not speak any English. Women like Bharti Hiram often felt extremely isolated because they had come to the UK alone to join husbands and families whom they did not know in advance: 'I'm just alone here. No-one here is my family, I'm the only one' (p.195).

Some carers feel that the only release from the burden of caring as they perceive it is with the death of those for whom they care. In a collection of the experiences of a number of carers, edited by Anna Briggs and Judith Oliver (1985), one woman in her late fifties, Doreen Hore, expressed it thus:

'Birth is a natural process. It can be planned and there is a time limit: not so with death. It may be taboo to discuss it, but the only ultimate release for the carer is the death of the patient' (p.79).

And in the same volume, another woman of similar age and circumstances voiced her fears about the future:

'Other days I'm the lonely clown trapped in a circus knowing there is another way of life on the outside but unable to escape and participate. When I look to the future I quell panic within. I am resigned to the fact that there is no way out. One day the caring will cease; the rigid routines will stop. What then? Will it be too late to build anything at all for myself. Will I be capable and able? If not, then who will care for the carer?' (p.104).

Another disturbing consequence of deteriorating family situations where elderly people and their relatives are thrown unwillingly together in the caring relationship are the instances of breakdown leading to abuse (Claudine Macreadie, 1991; Jackie Pritchard, 1992; Decalmer and Glendenning, in press; Bennett and Kingston, in press). The privacy of people's homes may sometimes mask acute misery, fear and pain. No one knows the extent to which 'elder abuse' takes place at home, but Eastman (1984) has estimated that 500 000 elderly people may be at risk from their own relatives. The Social Services Inspectorate (1992) describes the typical victim as white, female, over 75 years of age, with a physical or mental disability, who is living with an adult child. It is often easier to believe that ill-treatment only takes place in residential settings where people are being cared for by non-relatives; the idea of abuse by relatives in one's own home offends the ideal of the home as haven and refuge from a hostile outside world.

Differing perspectives: support for carers and care-recipients

Just as feminists have raised the issue of informal caring and the policy of community care in general during the past decade, so carers themselves have become vocal during the same period. As noted earlier, prior to this carers were barely seen as a separate, functioning category of the population. True, there was the National Council for the Single Woman and her Dependants, but this was generally regarded as a small interest group with little wider significance. It was concerned with a specific social issue, namely that of the single woman who either stayed at home, never going out to work, in order to care for an elderly parent, or who gave up work in mid-career to do so.

As care in the community became more of a public issue, carers began to see themselves as a group. In 1982, the Association of Carers was formed with the clear intention of bringing the concerns of carers to national prominence. During the past decade, carers have fought for society's recognition of the social and economic contribution which they make; they have campaigned for carers' benefits/wages and better support services, including day care and respite care (Jill Pitkeathley, 1991).

Government has responded in a limited way, often under pressure. For example, it has provided some funding for the Association of Carers (becoming the Carers National Association after its merger with the National Council for the Single Woman and her Dependants) which has been active in developing support networks for carers. It has also funded an information and support unit run by the King's Fund. The latter has been particularly active in developing guides for carers, training and resource material for health and social services staff and for establishing links with black and minority ethnic carers, through the production of videos and of information packs in relevant languages.

Government policy however has been to rely on informal care as

a core component of community care—and informal care, by definition, is cheap care, because it does not take account of the costs
absorbed by carers—a point which the Treasury is unlikely to have
overlooked. Government has not been prepared to put major
resources into the fundamental demands being made by carers. For
example, carers campaigned strenuously to have the 1975 Invalid
Care Allowance extended to married women. This was only conceded
as the result of a European Court ruling in 1986 (Hicks, 1988). Nor,
as yet, has there been any substantial increase in the basic level of
support services available in the community.

Elderly people form by far the largest client group served by community care policies and, in turn, form by far the largest group cared
for by informal carers. In theory, informal carers should be supported
by a range of statutory and voluntary services which should alleviate
some of the caring tasks (but does not remove the obligation—the
carer often has no choice as to whether to care or not). Moreover,
the ideological view that it is a woman's responsibility to care may
have practical consequences. Some of the tentative findings about
the differential levels of support that female and male carers receive
from the formal services points to this (Charlesworth *et al.*, 1984;
Mildred Blaxter, 1980): if a woman is caring then there is less need
to supply support services than if a man is caring (that is, one can
'manage', the other cannot). Indeed, 'some services state explicitly
in their policy documents that they do not provide a service to elderly
people who have female carers living in the vicinity' (Dee Jones,
1992, p.26). This situation is compounded for minority ethnic carers
who are often denied culturally sensitive help and whose acute lack
of knowledge about services stems from both barriers to communication and experiences of racism (Bould, 1990; McCalman, 1990).
Karl Atkin and his colleagues (1989) also found that, contrary to
widely held beliefs, Asian elders were only marginally less interested
in using services than their white counterparts.

In spite of recent legislation (the NHS and Community Care Act,
1990), which promises support for carers and those they care for,
it appears that resources will not be made available. Implementation
of the community care elements of the act has been delayed and,
in any case, critics have already said its intention is more about
rationing resources (through the assessment procedures vested in the
hands of local authorities which will act as gatekeepers to services)
than opening them up. As the numbers of elderly people (women in
particular) in the population grow and as competition for younger
women's labour increases, more and more older women, having given
a lifetime of caring themselves, will come to depend on the vagaries
of scarce formal services or on the compulsory altruism of informal
carers.

Discussion of the carer's perspective frequently tends to focus on the 'burden of caring'. This is perhaps inevitable since most organizations for carers aim to secure greater recognition and rights through campaigning; they are therefore bound to concentrate on the problems and difficulties which they face. But it is important to remember that there are other views. Many people in the disability movement reject the notion implicit in the arguments of carers that disabled people are the passive recipients of care and are therefore, of necessity, a burden on others. They turn the argument around. Far from disabled people themselves being a burden, society itself imposes a burden on them; they are disabled by a society which refuses to recognize their basic civil rights of equal recognition and access (Oliver, 1990). As Lois Keith (1990) has forcefully argued:

> 'In wanting to show how difficult and unrecognised the work of the carer is, many have thought it necessary to portray those who may be in need of care as passive, feeble and demanding. And so deep-rooted are our prejudices about both disabled and elderly people, that no-one really seems to have noticed the damage this can do. It merely confirms what most of us believe about disabled people anyway—that they are more or less helpless and need to be looked after by others. In this debate they are continuously presented as "the other", the non-person. They are rarely seen as having valuable lives in the way their able-bodied carer or partner does' (p.v).

Many disabled people thus reject the very concept of care, arguing that this implies merely the passive receipt of care from dominant able-bodied people (Wood, 1991). They favour the term 'support', or 'personal assistance', with the disabled person in control of what is offered and what is accepted. They argue very strongly for policies which would place money directly in the hands of disabled people to enable them to buy in the support services they identify for themselves as being necessary rather than being allocated services assessed as necessary by professional care workers.

Jenny Morris (1991), for example, adopts this view and criticizes feminist critics of community care who concentrate only on the impact the policies have on carers. She acknowledges the pressure on carers, often women, but argues that greater recognition should be given to the disabled woman's perspective. Feminists, she says, have separated disabled women off from other women and ignored them. Arguments against community care tend to concentrate on the burdens faced by women as carers and not on the pressures felt by women in receipt of informal care. Feminists, she goes on to argue, should be supporting and empowering disabled women in their struggle to live in the community on their own terms, in control of the support they need.

It is unfortunate that the interests of two groups of people, both oppressed by current social policies, should often seem to run counter to each other. Demands by one for greater support for carers

(Pitkeathley, 1991) is seen by the other as compounding social in-justice for disabled people (Wood, 1991). It is hard to see how these opposing views can be reconciled, although since both groups are disadvantaged by current policies, it would be in both their interests that some sort of reconciliation was reached. Perhaps alternatives to family-based models of care may need to be re-examined. Within the framework of community-care policies and the above debates within the disability movement these models have been rejected out of hand. Yet, if for the reasons explained earlier informal care itself is often unacceptable—because it imposes too great a burden on women (as carers and care-recipients) and because it represents an abdication of collective responsibility—then alternatives may have to be found. Institutional care, as it exists in many forms at present, may be anath-ema but there may be forms of residential or group care which can be established that avoid the isolation and fragmentation of com-munity care on the one hand and the 'warehousing' of the large institutions on the other (see pp.136–42).

Communities based on independent living principles for those who favour them, retirement 'villages' where elderly people maintain con-trol over their lives in a well-supported environment (which includes medical, nursing and social services), neighbourhood provision of day care and domiciliary services which are plentiful and accessible and linked with residential provision when required may be some of the ways forward. There may be lessons from Scandinavia and the USA and from the many other societies which are characterized by collective approaches to living and caring (Dalley, 1988). Currently, residential provision is stigmatized regardless of the standard of care provided. The 'policy fashion' which decries such forms of care has established a uniform and stereotyped view of it which is hard to contest. This has knock-on effects for people who in other circum-stances might think of looking on it more favourably. The challenge, therefore, for those who wish to devise alternatives to the narrow, individualistic forms of caring which presently prevail, is to persuade others to set aside those stereotyped attitudes.

Conclusion—Is there a way forward?

Community care, with its particular reliance on informal caring and family-based models of care, does not serve women well, whether they are care givers or receivers. Much of the philosophy behind community care in the early days was admirable—namely, its empha-sis on the rights of disabled people, of elderly people and of mentally ill people and of those with learning difficulties to lives of dignity and independence.

However, the original philosophy of community care which stresses independence, privacy, and self-help, along with models of care based on the family, have become inextricably bound up with the ideology of individualism. This has fuelled social welfare policy in recent years (Dalley, 1988). It reasserts the responsibility of individuals and their families to care for themselves; it argues against what has come to be known as the 'culture of dependency', suggesting that the state provision of services to people in need has a debilitating effect on them. People should fend for themselves wherever possible. In spite of four decades of the welfare state, policy is now based on a view that the state's appropriate role in the provision of welfare should be a residual one (Green, 1992). Individualist ideology centres on individual liberty, competition and the market. Vulnerable people will benefit from the 'tenderness' of those who succeed in the competitive environment of the market (Joseph and Sumption, 1979). Thus the provision of welfare will ultimately depend on the charitable 'do-gooding' concern of the free and the powerful. The dependent and the powerless will have little say in shaping their own fate; they will have to rely on charity and voluntary action (Plant, 1985).

There has thus been a convergence between two sets of ideas. On the one hand, there was the early thinking behind community care which stressed notions of independence and the view that the appropriate location for care is within the family. On the other is individualism which, because of a belief in the all-pervading superiority of reliance on the market as a means of social regulation, stresses the responsibility of families to provide and underplays any collective responsibility on the part of the state or society at large. Opponents would argue that this is unacceptable and that concepts of reciprocity, fellowship and cooperation are better values on which to base a community-care strategy than the rugged, individualistic competition of the market.

This chapter has suggested that the welfare of many people, particularly elderly people, has come to depend on the altruistic commitment of informal carers, the majority of whom are women. In turn, women themselves as they grow older become the chief recipients of informal care—or, perhaps, of no care at all. Moreover, this altruistic commitment has been coopted into supporting the ideology of individualism that has informed social welfare policy in recent years. Sadly, the admirable impulses that individuals have in caring for their dependants are turned in on themselves rather than being subsumed into a wider ethos of social responsibility across society.

We argue that it is necessary to call upon a different ideological view if a more equitable solution is to be found—both for women and those for whom they care. Collective approaches to the tasks of caring, it is argued, are more likely to devise solutions which do not depend on the compulsory altruism of women and which do not force disabled and frail people into unacceptable relationships of dependency on relatives and friends or into lives of isolation and loneliness.

7 The living environments of older women

Sheila Peace

'. . . I quite like living alone, I don't have to tell anybody what I'm going to do next, making decisions, and carrying them out. I wouldn't like it if I didn't ever see anybody . . . Looking around, I think I'll stay until I—I'd sooner put up with the disadvantages of—um—I don't like the idea of being in a home. But I don't think I want to live with any of my children completely, either. I don't think too much about it. I mean this works, I've got a small flat, which I can manage. And unless something disastrous happens to me I think I could manage for a reasonably long time.'

(Joan)

Introduction: women and spatial relations

The quality of our environment is an important facet of our quality of life (Beverley Hughes, 1990). The need for shelter is a basic human need and our desire for a secure habitat from which to conduct our lives is fundamental. This chapter is primarily concerned with women's needs in terms of accommodation in later life. But to understand these needs we must consider a number of wider issues, in particular the importance of home and community in shaping women's lives and how they may help us understand some of the decisions which older women have to face regarding where they live at the end of their lives.

The importance of gender to our understanding of spatial relations, especially within the urban environment, has gone unrecognized until relatively recently. The work of feminist writers from a number of disciplines has drawn our attention to a range of issues. Of most importance are: the ideologies surrounding home and community; the importance of the family as a unit of production and consumption; the separation and integration of the private and the public spheres; the inequalities experienced by many women in relation to housing; the role of women within the housing professions; and how housing design has reflected and reinforced popular assumptions about gender differences (Leonore Davidoff *et al.*, 1976; Marion Brion and Anthea Tinker, 1980; Linda McDowell, 1983; Matrix, 1984; Jo Little *et al.*, 1988). These are the issues which form the starting point for this chapter.

Home and community

It would seem crucial that we should focus first on home and community. The view that 'woman's place is in the home' has been, and remains, a very powerful image within our society. So too is the notion that the local community or neighbourhood is a place for women's activity. They are both seen as 'good things', and there is a sense that without both home and community, society will in some ways disintegrate into an unruly mess. But where did these ideals originate and how have they survived? Leonore Davidoff and her colleagues (1976) provide a thought-provoking account of how, since pre-industrial times, home and rural village community have been idealized and utilized in order to maintain a set of power relations between both men and women and between different classes within society. They argue that within the community and the home, symbolic boundaries were established so that those with power could limit access to a broader range of experience for those seen as subordinate in terms of class or gender.

Our views have been developed within a paternalistic, patriarchal society where the home is seen as the embodiment of family life. The home then has been idealized as a domestic idyll and is the basis for family reproduction, production and consumption—all areas where women play an important role.

Throughout the nineteenth and twentieth centuries the planning and design of settlements reinforced these ideals. The development of planned communities, such as the 'garden city movement', all served to enhance a separation of the spheres of domestic (unpaid) and paid labour and to reinforce the notions of public and private lives which often came to be equated with men and women. Thus, the home and the local community were essentially seen as the locus of domestic life while workers travelled away from home to their place of paid employment (McDowell, 1983).

While attention has focused in recent years on the private lives of women and the unseen unpaid labour of domestic life (Ann Oakley, 1976), we have also become conscious of the way in which the public and private spheres of life for women are no longer separate; more often than not they are highly integrated (MacKenzie, 1988). Women with dual roles, who juggle the responsibilities for paid work with the demands of family care, are beginning to redefine their use of both time and space. Thus, the mother with a full-time job and children of school age has to find alternative after-school care which may be outside the family home, and the daughter with a part-time job who also cares for her elderly mother, but who lives at a distance, has to combine trips with phone calls and the support of neighbours and statutory services.

Focusing on these issues leads us to ask who it is who actually lives within the home and what does it look like? A common ideal of the twentieth century is of the nuclear family with husband and wife and two children occupying a two- or three-bedroom house. Yet this is an inaccurate reflection of current society, with 60 per cent of households no longer meeting this model (Jos Boys *et al.*, 1984). The days of the extended family with several generations occupying the same unit of accommodation are also no longer common, although such arrangements are more frequent amongst some ethnic groups within the UK.

The importance of design

It is common to think of the home as a very private place. Indeed, in terms of family life it is true to say that once inside the front door much of what goes on is invisible. Jos Boys and her colleagues (1984), in their enlightening discussion of housing design and women's roles show how, from the early nineteenth century onwards, house design has increasingly come to embody the 'privatization of family life'. During the course of the twentieth century the demise of live-in domestic labour and the growth of labour-saving devices placed more and more emphasis on the woman's role within the home for all sectors of society. In 1918, the Tudor Walters Committee, set up to look at new methods of building houses for the working classes, heard evidence from the Women's Housing Sub-Committee which had canvassed the views of working-class women living on housing estates. Amongst their demands were:

> 'a separate workroom for cooking and food preparation; a separate bathroom; a front parlour; labour-saving devices (such as hot and cold running water, a kitchen range which did not involve stooping, with easy clean finishes); and play spaces for both older and younger children' (Barbara McFarlane, 1984, p.29).

The recommendations of the Tudor Walters Committee set many of the standards for municipal suburban houses throughout the 1920s, 1930s and 1940s. Two factors became dominant. First, that the model for housing was the nuclear family and second, that the wife's role was to carry out all the domestic work within the home.

The maintenance of this dominant ideology of the home as 'women's place' continued during the postwar period. It was not until the 1960s that planning guidance began to reflect something of the diversity of living arrangements. The 1961 Parker Morris Report 'Homes for Today and Tomorrow' recognized the 'greater demand by single people for separate houses rather than living with their families or as lodgers, and the need for housing to provide more than a minimal "roof over the head"—to cater for a collection of individuals with aspirations and with differing and sometimes conflicting interests' (Boys *et al.*, 1984, p.78). While the recognition of such diversity led to recommendations for more space and heating in bedrooms to allow use during the day, in general the design of houses still perpetuated the traditional picture of the nuclear family, with a clear division between male and female roles.

This discussion of the ideology of home and community, which has been reinforced by the design and planning of predominantly family-oriented housing and community facilities, is fundamental to our understanding of the experiences of living arrangements that women bring with them to later life. It also underpins the meaning of home for older people within our society.

Home and self-identity in later life

Home can be viewed from a number of different perspectives—physical, material, social and psychological—each of which may have a different meaning for older people. In the physical sense, home is defensible space. But the control of this defensible space may differ in relation to gender and across the life course. How easy is it to permit or deny access to our home in later life, and how far do people remain in control?

At a material level the acquisition of objects within the home may lead to a level of possessiveness. However, this also enables us to develop a familiarity with our environment which is reinforced through memories that help us to connect the past with the present. As a social setting home also means people, family, and pets, and even though many older people live alone and experience reduced social networks, research shows that they still retain links with their community which enable them to maintain an important sense of self-identity through an association with place (Sarah Matthews, 1979; Sandra Howell, 1983; Rowles, 1983).

Older people are often said to be attached to their homes, and this attachment is shown in both their unusually long residence in a single location and the desire of the majority to live out their lives at home. Studies of older people's satisfaction with their housing point to the complexity of the topic: people want to stay put because home has associations with family and related memories, something particularly true for older women; they feel competent in a familiar environment where disability is accepted; the status of home ownership may give them a sense of control in a world which devalues them, and they find that some of the disadvantages of remaining at home are outweighed by the advantages (Golant, 1982; Shirley O'Bryant, 1983; Sixsmith, 1986).

The importance of home as a power base is echoed in the sense of 'competence', 'value' and 'status' which may be achieved by living in a familiar environment. But do accommodation needs change in later life? Here the concepts of 'environmental congruence' and 'environmental press' are useful (M. Powell Lawton and Lucy Nahemow, 1973; Lawton, 1980; Sheila Peace, 1988). It can be argued that throughout our lives we try to maintain 'environmental congruence'—that is we try, given the resources available to us, to adapt our habitat to meet our needs. However, at any time our needs may fall out of step with our environment, leading to 'environmental press', and we may not have the material resources to change our surroundings. The circumstances of ownership of property may not allow for adaptation. We may not be physically competent; we may lack the necessary skills to make such adaptations, and help may not be readily available. In addition we may feel insecure in our environment, since the community in which we live may have changed or feel hostile towards us.

At one level we might use this model to suggest that some older people affected by increasingly frail health and reduced resources may need to live in a more supportive environment as they get older. But there is also an argument (Lawton, 1983) that a certain level of 'environmental press' can create tensions through which the individual may continue to master their environment. This may be the reason why many older people choose to go on living in accommodation which appears not to meet their needs, while others living in institutional settings become apathetic and inactive. The importance of a familiar environment in maintaining self-identity cannot be overlooked when considering accommodation in later life, and the trauma of moving can be particularly painful for some (Audrey McCollum, 1990).

Home and homeland

Age, sex, race and class are all important in helping us understand the value of attachment to place throughout the life course (Redfoot and Black, 1988). Here we should also recognize the differing perspectives on home and homeland experienced by older people from black and minority ethnic groups in the UK. Research has shown that amongst some older Afro-Caribbeans there is still a longing to return to their homeland, and that while there may be an acceptance that this will not become a reality, it is still a fondly held dream (Fenton, 1987).

However, it appears that this view of homeland is not universal amongst older people from minority ethnic groups. It was not a view expressed by those older people from South Asian communities to whom Fenton spoke in Bristol (1987). For these people, home and the family group meant security, and their main concerns were about insecurity and isolation in old age, often due to their lack of understanding of the English language and their fear of racial attacks within the home (Alison Norman, 1985). For many, their families are now settled in the UK. In a small study based on the oral histories of 10 older Afro-Caribbean women, Gwen Caesar (1987) shows how women are often acutely aware of how things may have changed 'at home'. One woman says:

> 'I've got to stay here, it's cheaper and any way what are you going to do. The people you knew are all dead now and it's just the young and they don't have time for you' (p.53).

Consequently, while some of the facets of home and its meaning may be common to all older people, we should recognize the diversity of meanings which exist and the variety of experiences which underpin older women's current living arrangements.

Where older women live—the diversity of experience

People over 75 years of age and those living alone (the majority of whom are women) are just as likely to be found living in declining industrial areas and the inner cities as in coastal retirement towns and inland rural areas of England and Wales (Warnes and Law, 1985). Differences in distribution reflect a number of factors, most notably the development of retirement areas; the out-migration of the young from rural communities, older industrial areas and inner cities; the historical in-migration of ethnic groups; and the *in situ* ageing of particular populations. All of these may in turn have a bearing on issues of a more local or personal nature such as the proximity of family and friends; the availability of small units of manageable housing, and access to local systems of support.

Since the Second World War the number of older people who own their own home has increased. Current figures show that nearly half of older heads of household are owner-occupiers. However, definitions of head of household, which give precedence to males over females, make our interpretation of figures with regard to older women problematic. For example, we have no real information concerning the numbers of married older women who jointly own property with their husbands. In the 1988 GHS (OPCS, 1990d) figures are given for tenure by sex and marital status. This indicates that 43 per cent of widowed females are outright owner-occupiers, 45 per cent rent from either local authority/new town or housing association/cooperative, and 8 per cent live in private rented, unfurnished accommodation. We therefore need to look at a range of housing tenures when considering women's experiences of housing.

For older people from black and minority ethnic groups, the data suggests that a large majority of Asian households are likely to be living in owner-occupied property, while Afro-Caribbean households are more evenly split between owner-occupied and local authority accommodation (OPCS, 1990d). These patterns of accommodation reflect different historical phases of immigration, and the experiences of male immigrants whose families often joined them at a later date (Sheila Mackintosh *et al.*, 1990). Some of the older black women interviewed by Caesar (1987) revealed the important relation which existed for many of those newly arrived in this country between finding a job and finding accommodation. One woman said: 'I couldn't afford a house, not even one room, so I shared with a friend when I first came over here' (p.32).

The experience of living alone may be less common amongst older women from black and minority ethnic communities. While the patterns of living arrangements associated with the extended family may be changing, there are distinct differences between ethnic groups (Fenton, 1987). Asian older people, for example, are more likely to live in large households than older Afro-Caribbeans, and amongst the Asian community, Pakistani and Bangladeshi families are now experiencing most overcrowding in terms of accommodation (OPCS, 1990c; CSO, 1991).

The importance for older people of the relation between income, housing tenure and housing conditions is currently receiving more attention (Mackintosh *et al.*, 1990; Christine Oldman, 1990). Successive English House Condition Surveys (EHCS) by the Department of the Environment (1983; 1988) have shown that older people are more likely than younger people to live in properties which lack basic amenities, are unfit, or are in disrepair, and this is particularly true of owner-occupied property and private rented accommodation (Mackintosh *et al.*, 1990). Given the number of older women living alone within both these types of property, this statement causes alarm.

In Chapter 3 of this book, Dulcie Groves explores the financial resources of older women and discusses the reasons why many of them experience extreme poverty. In terms of housing needs it is often those with the least resources who have the most need, and this is particularly true of those living alone. While income may decline on the death of a spouse, household bills do not, and increasing frailty may lead to a greater need for a warm home that is easy to get around and manage. Many older women who have been economically dependent on their spouse have to cope with housing responsibilities for the first time in their lives following his death.

Current issues in older women's experience of home and community

Although older women live in a wide range of different types of accommodation it is possible to highlight a number of common concerns which affect them all. In the discussion which follows, we shall look in more detail at 'resource issues', 'accommodation plus care', 'the relationship between home and community' and 'design issues'.

Resource issues: asset or liability?

We have already noted that there has been a rapid increase in owner-occupation throughout the twentieth century which looks likely to continue, and that the majority of households where the head is over retirement age now own their own home, and own it outright with no mortgage left to pay off (Mackintosh *et al.*, 1990). Amongst women currently in their sixties and seventies, a high proportion will experience owner-occupation as part of a married couple. And yet, a substantial minority of widowed and never-married women are also outright owner-occupiers, so living in owner-occupied accommodation and all the responsibilities this entails is central to many older women's lives.

What then are the main issues facing them? A major concern is 'does their accommodation meet their needs?' and 'can it be altered to meet changing needs?' This relates to the condition of the housing and whether the older person has the resources, both financial and personal, to maintain their property or to move to alternative accommodation such as a bungalow, flat or sheltered accommodation. A second issue, intimately connected with the first, concerns how owner-occupied property can be used as an asset in later life to fund accommodation plus care, and the impact this will have on the transfer of property between generations and the inheritance of wealth.

Where the maintenance of property is concerned we have seen that older people are likely to live in some of the least well-maintained accommodation, and that owner-occupied property needs some of the most costly repairs. A great deal has now been written on how people can be helped to maintain and repair their property (Rose Wheeler, 1985; Leather *et al.*, 1985), and Sheila Mackintosh and her colleagues (1990) provide a useful summary. The aim here then is not to repeat this material but to think about what it means for older women.

Many elderly home-owners want to stay in their own home for as long as possible, but have difficulty arranging and paying for repairs and maintenance. For many older women, they may feel further disadvantaged by their lack of knowledge and skill in this area. Dealing with household maintenance and repairs, especially major external repairs, has traditionally been seen as part of the male preserve —whether the husband, the male relative, neighbour or workman. Nevertheless, whereas this may mean that older women living alone may be more likely to neglect such necessary tasks, it is often not so much the organization of such work as the financing that holds people back, and as we have seen older women form some of the poorest households. What many people need is easily accessible advice and information, and 'Staying Put' schemes and 'Care and Repair' schemes do exist to assist older owner-occupiers (Karen Smith, 1988a). There are also a number of options available to help people raise money to pay for repairs. Some are entitled to improvement grants, currently administered by the local authorities. However the asset of owner-occupied property makes many people ineligible for these schemes. They become what Julie Bull and Lindsay Poole (1989) have called 'house rich, income poor', one of a number who occupy the middle ground of being 'not rich, not poor'—as this example indicates:

> 'Mrs C is an 80 year old widow who receives a state pension plus an occupational pension of £31.83 per month so she is not in receipt of Income Support. She needs to finance essential repairs, the cost of which will be around £10,000. Her house was built after 1919 so she is not eligible for a local authority grant. She feels that the repayment of interest on a maturity loan would not be affordable on her limited income. Her local care and repair scheme are finding it difficult to help Mrs C' (p.45).

The equity held in property varies widely according to the condition of the property, size, location and region of the country. Nevertheless, those with housing equity may be able to raise money by borrowing and using the outstanding equity in their property as security. A range of schemes are now becoming available: second mortgages, maturity loans, Home Income Plans and rolled-up interest loans (Mackintosh *et al.*, 1990). In many cases however the current generation of older women have not been involved in dealing with housing finances: they have not paid the mortgage or dealt with the building society or bank regarding such matters, and they may not know where to start. This is another reason why easy access to sound advice is a priority.

This argument also applies to issues concerning inheritance. The passing on of wealth between generations through the inheritance of property has in the past been seen as a way for wealthier groups within society to retain power and privilege (Engels, 1884; Janet

Finch, 1989). Today, with the rise in owner-occupation, this is becoming more of a commonplace within families, and the rights of individuals to dispose of their assets as they wish can take on a new significance (Finch, 1989). Married women therefore need to secure their right to inherit the family home through joint ownership, or provisions made in wills to which they are a party. Where divorce or separation increase the potential claimants to family property, it is particularly important that older women have safeguards against the possibility of becoming homeless.

Of course, the upkeep of property including gardens, the suitability and adaptability of accommodation and the need for sound advice and information are not only of concern for the owner-occupier. For those in private rented accommodation the poor condition of property can be particularly onerous. Problems often exist in getting landlords to undertake repairs and many tenants feel unable to complain about conditions for fear of harassment. In Karen Smith's study of the housing conditions of elderly private tenants in Kensington and Chelsea (1988b), she identifies the following areas as being particularly problematic: lack of knowledge regarding the rights of private tenants; the isolation of liaising with landlords on an individual basis; problems of disrepair; security of tenure; income difficulties; long-term residence coupled with declining health and inappropriate accommodation. She concludes that: 'For the vast majority of elderly private tenants there is no financial choice other than to stay put in the private rented sector' (pp.13–14).

Renting accommodation in the public sector or through Housing Associations presents older people with other concerns. The total stock of local authority housing has declined during the 1980s. Significant factors include a lack of investment in maintenance and new building, as well as the 'Right to Buy' movement. Despite this, older people still remain overrepresented within this sector. Tenants are likely to live in a variety of housing, such as tower blocks, flats in maisonette blocks, bungalows and two- or three-bedroom houses, while the number living in sheltered housing or other specialist accommodation remains relatively small (Mackintosh *et al.*, 1990). Many older people therefore occupy ordinary housing which may not be adapted for them. Living in accommodation which may not meet their needs is a reality for women living in both the public or private sectors.

All of those older women renting accommodation will also be affected by recent changes in the Housing Laws. The 1988 Housing Act relaxed rent controls on new lettings by private landlords and Housing Associations. While existing renters may retain their present rent arrangements, rents can be expected to rise following vacancies. In the private sector it is also more likely that property will continue to be sold into owner-occupation. Housing Associations will become a more important source of accommodation for older people, even though financing new projects remains difficult.

For council tenants, the new laws mean that they have the right under Tenants' Choice to transfer to Housing Associations, co-operatives or private landlords. Indeed, in some inner-city areas, Housing Action Trusts (HATs) are taking over council housing, reno-vating property, and then selling it to a variety of landlords. Local authorities have been actively discouraged from building more new housing for rent and manage less property than in the past. The lower rents experienced by many council tenants are also likely to become a thing of the past as new systems are introduced for deciding on 'fair' rents. As Mackintosh and her colleagues (1990) state: 'all elderly council house residents face the prospect of increased rents and a greater reliance upon the housing benefit system' (p.82). Indeed, in all sectors rent payments are likely to form a greater part of the older person's current expenditure, especially those who fail to qualify for housing benefits.

Accommodation plus care

For those older women who do not wish to or cannot 'stay put' in their current accommodation, what are the options? The obvious solution is to move, but to where? As we have seen, moving house in later life can be traumatic for some, especially for those women who may have made a great emotional investment in their home. In this section we look more closely at sheltered housing and residential care as two forms of accommodation which also incorporate an element of care. Although occupied by a very small proportion of all older people (i.e. sheltered housing: 5 per cent of those over retirement age; residential care: 4–6 per cent), they are of particular importance to the older frailer members of our society, and conse-quently become the domains of older women.

A range of options for moving in later life may be available for those with sufficient resources. Some owner-occupiers will trade down to a smaller more manageable bungalow or flat; others may opt for what is seen as more specialized accommodation—low-cost ownership schemes (Oldman, 1990), or sheltered housing provided by a local authority, Housing Association or private developer. For those pre-viously renting accommodation the options are rather more limited.

Sheltered housing

The majority of sheltered schemes offer flat-type accommodation exclusively for elderly people, with a common room and other shared facilities. Support is usually available from a warden backed by com-munications systems, usually alarms, for summoning assistance in emergencies. While the early provision was made primarily by the local authorities, over time there has been a diversification of schemes with the involvement of Housing Associations and private developers. Oldman puts the number of sheltered housing units at the end of 1989 in the region of 500 000 in England and Wales, of which 50 000 are in the private sector (1990, p.23). However, regional distribution of all sheltered schemes is very uneven.

Sheltered housing has also become a particularly important housing alternative for older people from minority ethnic groups. Loss of family support coupled with social isolation and the fear of racial harassment has made sheltered housing a particularly attractive option for many groups (Alison Norman, 1985; Voluntary Housing, 1987). In particular, it can provide an environment which is designed to meet the cultural needs and customs of the users. A sheltered housing scheme can become a focal part of a wider community, with well-used communal areas and wardens with particular skills in terms of language and understanding. During the 1980s a number of Housing Associations, or groups within already established Housing Associations, emerged and began to develop such schemes, e.g. Asian Sheltered Residential Accommodation (ASRA), Carib Housing Association, Jewish Welfare Board. The emergence of special provision for those from minority ethnic groups may also be seen as the only option in a system which does not address their needs. Caesar (1987) comments:

> 'The possibility of qualifying for housing association homes or sheltered accommodation is confounded by the priorities that these organisations set themselves. For example, young families with children rather than one elderly person is seen to be more of a priority. One woman knew of a sheltered housing scheme near her but says, There is only one black person there. I don't expect they'll want anymore' (p.42).

In recent years there has also been a general move towards providing very sheltered housing or 'extra care' facilities where support services and higher levels of staffing are offered as a way of maintaining more dependent older people within what has traditionally been seen as 'housing' rather than 'residential care'. Since 1984, such schemes run by Housing Associations and the private sector have been able to register under the Registered Homes Act 1984, and to take advantage of board and lodgings income support payments for low income tenants (Tinker, 1989). These developments have fuelled the debate over the nature and role of sheltered housing. Do such schemes offer housing or social support, or both? Traditionally run via housing departments and housing agencies, sheltered housing has sought to maintain the control of the householder over their property. Thus individuals buy or rent their accommodation and maintain relatively 'private lives'. Yet some would argue that what sheltered housing

dwellers value most of all is modern, well-maintained, secure housing, and that this need not necessarily be provided in age-segregated
complexes (Oldman, 1990; Wheeler, 1986; Laura Middleton, 1987).
What is needed is more housing options. Others however, point to
the changing characteristics and needs of sheltered housing dwellers
who, as they get older, frailer and more in need of social support,
are more likely to value the warden service with its ability to mobilize
help in emergencies (Fennell, 1986; Fennell *et al.*, 1988).

For those buying into the growing private sheltered housing
market, the issues of accommodation and care are perhaps more
starkly bound up with housing finance. Buying into such a property
is commonly accompanied by service charges which may initially
relate only to repair and maintenance but gradually come to include
hotel and care costs. For older women on fixed incomes their ability
to pay for their accommodation plus care can become increasingly
burdensome (Fleiss, 1985).

What then do we know of the women who form the majority of
occupants in such schemes? Research by Fennell (1986) in schemes
run by the Anchor Housing Association and by Williams (1990) in
private for sale and leasehold schemes show that all tenants have
some remarkably similar characteristics. They are predominantly
female, living in single-person households and with an average age
in the mid 70s. They also commonly lack social support. In the study
by Williams one-quarter of his respondents (n = 515) were childless
and a further 25 per cent had only one child. Lack of access to family
support was therefore an important consideration in moving to such
accommodation.

There were also important differences. In the Anchor study (Fennell, 1986), while the majority felt they were relatively independent,
they were more likely than the general elderly population to experience falls, illness and disability. More than one-quarter of the Anchor
tenants had found it necessary to summon help in an emergency
within the 12 months prior to the study—with falls being the most
common reason (Fennell, 1986). In contrast, Williams' respondents
(1990) were more likely to be in upper income groups, with the
majority from non-manual backgrounds. They appeared to be a much
fitter group than the general elderly population, a factor which the
author discusses in relation to the screening procedures undertaken
by many of the private developments. The respondents showed a
remarkably low level of take-up of health and welfare services. They
had chosen to move into special accommodation because it provided
a smaller more manageable property, which offered security and the
comfort of a warden service, was often in close proximity to family
or friends, offered a peer group of their own age and was in easy
access of shops and communal facilities. Data such as these begin to
tell us something of the different characteristics of older people in

the various sectors of specialist housing and the subtle differences which exist in the continuum of need for accommodation plus care.

Residential care

If sheltered housing has had a predominantly 'good press' with older people and their relatives, then residential care has to be seen as its antithesis. Yet the world of residential care for older people is truly a woman's world: over three-quarters of residents are women and the majority are over 85 years of age. A recent government statistical report by the Department of Health (1991) comments:

> 'In the under-65 age group the numbers of male and female residents is almost equal. The ratio gradually increases with age until there are almost six times as many female residents as male residents aged 85 and over. This trend can be seen throughout the residential population of elderly people. This is not simply due to demographic factors as female residents account for a greater proportion of the total female population aged 85 and over than do male residents in equivalent age groups. The effect may be due to a higher proportion of elderly men with a living spouse and a lower proportion living alone' (para 2.4).

Marital status compounds the picture and shows for example that never-married women in their late seventies are eight times more likely than married women of the same age to find themselves in residential care (Sara Arber and Jay Ginn, 1991b). This and other research has shown that residents are predominantly widowed and never-married females in their late eighties, and that a large proportion have lived alone prior to admission (Sinclair, 1988). Admission to residential care has often come after a period in hospital, but for those admitted from the community, ill health coupled with either their own or a carer's inability to cope are key factors in the decision to accept a residential place.

Data show that whereas in 1976 72 per cent of residents were accommodated in the public sector facilities, 13 per cent in the voluntary sector and only 11 per cent in the private sector, by 1988 these percentages had been transformed into 45 per cent, 11 per cent and 44 per cent, respectively (Mackintosh *et al.*, 1990). What is even more dramatic, however, is the regional diversity in the proportion of people over 85 years living in residential accommodation, with higher than average percentages in areas such as Devon, Clwyd, the Isle of Wight, East and West Sussex, Warwickshire and North Yorkshire. Given that many of these parts of the country contain retirement areas it may be the case that where intensive family support is scarce, and where alternative living environments are more common, a residential lifestyle may become more acceptable or more essential (Peace, 1987).

If residential care is becoming a more common experience for women in very old age, what do we know of their experience? While much research has been undertaken in residential care, to date there remains a dearth of research differentiating between the experiences of men and women. Dianne Willcocks and her colleagues (1982; 1987), using material from a large national consumer study of residents of 100 local authority old people's homes, began to highlight some of the differences. In particular they showed how women were more likely to lose control over their admission to a residential home, events often resulting in the intervention of a 'third party' such as a GP or social worker. This point is reflected in the experience of Mrs Mullard, one of those women interviewed by Janet Ford and Ruth Sinclair (1987). She had been living with her son and his wife prior to moving into a residential home.

> 'I used to go to Faringdon House on a Wednesday and I'd been to one or two places for a fortnight while they'd been on their holidays. One time I'd been here. In the end they said I'd be better looked after, so when it was decided I'd move for good I said I'd come here, but I wish I hadn't done . . . Now if anyone asks me I always say that if you can keep your own home it's best to do so as long as possible because however nice a place is it's not like home is it? When you're at home you can do as you like, although when you get as you can't manage you've got to go somewhere like this' (p.33).

For those moving into private residential care it may be thought that 'paying for your care' would give you greater control over your life. However, recent research by Isobel Allen and her colleagues (1992) shows little difference in the consumer power and influence exerted by female residents for either public or private sector residential homes. Many of the women interviewed in private residential homes had their finances managed by other members of their family, often a son, and concerns were more likely to be about managing increasing fees on a fixed income.

While losing personal control over admission to a residential care home is one form of loss, researchers have also demonstrated how the residential lifestyle may also depersonalize individuals, and that this may be more true for one of the majority of women than for one of the minority of men. Again, as Dianne Willcocks (1986) observes:

> 'the acceptance of domestic and physical care by a group of predominantly female staff represents no major threat to men who achieve a relatively high degree of control and satisfaction in residential settings. In contrast, women who enter care are generally older, less fit and have fewer resources to enable them to adjust to the strangeness of receiving care, after accumulated experience of offering care to others. Identity and self-esteem may suffer with removal from the intimate domestic sphere of their former home. It is a substantial indictment of residential care that

the life style is not designed to satisfy the needs of this majority group' (p.151).

In the National Consumer Study mentioned above, the development of what the authors termed 'residential flatlets' (Willcocks *et al.*, 1982; 1987) was seen as one way of refocusing residential life around the needs of the individual within a collective setting. The recommendations of the Wagner Committee, whose review of residential care in 1988 supported the view that accommodation and care must be seen as separate but linked areas of need, should be implemented (National Institute for Social Work, 1988). Certainly the debate over how best we can combine our needs for a 'home' and our needs for care in later life must be continued (Finch, 1984; Gillian Dalley, 1988; Jenny Morris, 1992). We need to hear more of the views of older women about the advantages and disadvantages of different styles of living, whether in collective or family settings. And within special settings we need to recognize that the dividing lines between sheltered housing, residential homes and nursing homes can be very fine. More thought should be given as to how we have managed to forget, by compartmentalizing each within their own organizational boundaries, that people seek measures of flexibility in their need for accommodation plus care.

To summarize, the housing system in this country, based as it is on the importance of private property and private family life, forces on many older women either 'individual or family-based' solutions to their needs or the option of a more 'institutional' solution. And therein lies the dilemma. In both cases the older woman may find herself living an isolated existence. The ideology of 'community care' (see Chapter 6), based on the premise that older people should be enabled to remain in their own homes for as long as possible, in many ways reinforces this division. Living in ordinary housing in the community is what most older people say they want, but with increasingly poor health and without family or community support this may be far from their ideal. Such a view is reflected in this comment from an 82-year-old woman living in a residential care home interviewed in the study by Allen *et al.* (1992):

'I just couldn't cope with it. I couldn't live at home. Those empty houses outside each side; they all went to work and I did not say anything to anyone. I was so lonely. Just so fed up and on my own. Here it's company . . .' (p.166).

Alternative housing options need to be explored. The ideas found within collective or communal living, of shared responsibility, as yet have found little support, and while examples do exist in this country such as in Abbeyfield Houses or the Bexley Home Share Scheme or family placement schemes, they remain small-scale initiatives for a minority compared to the housing experiences of the majority (Sheila Peace and Charlotte Nusberg, 1984; Nan Maitland, 1991).

Bringing home and community together

While accommodation and housing circumstances form the main focus of this chapter, we began by setting the home within the community. We noted that the local community has been viewed traditionally as a woman's place, a place for shopping, meeting friends and neighbours, where children have grown up and gone to school, a place of familiar networks. What then are the issues concerning the wider community for women as they age?

Moving about the community means crossing the threshold of that private space 'home' into the semiprivate/public and public areas which surround it. While the garden or the yard may feel like safe territory, the alley, the courtyard and the street may feel more dangerous places for a woman, and especially as she ages and may experience a loss of mobility. Mrs Harman, one of the women interviewed by Ford and Sinclair (1987) expresses her feelings on the subject:

'I don't like stopping in during the day. I say to myself, Oh go out while you've got the chance: you never know what's in front of you, so I'll go into town, and to a club one afternoon, or for a walk, or to work in the garden. But I don't go out at night—no, I stop at home every evening. I won't go out in the dark—I'd be afraid . . . I think the older you get you do feel more nervous really, and I don't think it's because we've talked ourselves into it; I think there really is danger out there—when you hear of some of what these youths do, snatching handbags and all that' (p.26).

This sense of vulnerability needs to be acknowledged and challenged. Women need to feel safer within their own environment at all times (see p.164).

Women, particularly those of the current older generations, have less access to a car and are less likely to have learned to drive (Laurie Pickup, 1988). Consequently, under their own steam they may find themselves restricted to their locality (Stuart, 1991). As a result public transport can take on a greater significance. But its cost, availability and ease of access can vary widely between areas (Oxley, 1989). Enormous differences exist between the availability of transport in rural and urban areas; in some parts of the country concessionary fares operate for older people, while in others they are non-existent (O'Reilly, 1988), and even fewer examples can be found of authorities who have experimented with easier physical access to transport (Oxley and Benwell, 1989).

We need to think again about what we mean by 'the importance of local facilities'—a phase often found in planning documents regarding specialist accommodation and facilities for older people. If we think of shopping as an example of one of the most frequent reasons for women to make trips within their community, then the key issues here are access, transport, safety and comfort. The corner shop may score on proximity but may prove expensive and difficult to negotiate with a shopping trolley. More thought needs to be given as to how older people can be enabled to carry on with their daily activities for as long as possible. Is there a role for more mobile services within the community? Being able to take part in our local community is important for maintaining our self-esteem, and lessons need to be learnt about the poor location of facilities; the cracked and raised pavements that are hazardous to those whose mobility is poor; the taxicard services that only a few people know about.

The restrictions on lifestyle caused by environments that fail to recognize the needs of all users has been commented on repeatedly, and yet very little is done to rectify the situation. Such matters have become important campaigning issues for some groups of older people (for example the fight in London to preserve the free bus pass) but they have only just begun to scratch the surface of this important area.

Design issues

In this chapter we have also seen how both the form and the function of housing have played important roles in shaping and moulding women's lives. In later life then, it is not surprising that women have things to say about the design of their home and community. In relation to sheltered housing and residential care, we find that in terms of the overall size of care settings, 'small is beautiful'. Williams' respondents (1990) in private sheltered housing expressed lower satisfaction with their accommodation when schemes became too large (mean size: 35 units; range: 14–76 units), and Willcocks et al. (1987) show that complex design layouts in residential homes often prove confusing to many residents. Where internal design is concerned the issues are numerous. Again Williams' respondents mentioned the poor quality of lighting, the inadequacy of laundry areas, the lack of handrail supports, dark lifts and corridors, the small dimensions of living rooms and the dislike of an open-plan lounge/kitchen arrangement, the poor location of electric sockets, inadequate storage space, and the height and depth of baths. For those respondents in the 1981 National Consumer Study of Local Authority Homes (Willcocks et al., 1982; 1987), the request was more basic—having 'a room of my own' was one of the most important messages here, which while adhered to in many residential and nursing homes is still not an option for all residents.

A recent study by the Women's Design Service (1991) gathered evidence from a smaller number of older women in a range of housing types. The authors discuss nine areas that were of most concern to those interviewed: affordability; issues relating to mobility and disability; health and support services; caring (and design issues); comfort; safety; security; domestic violence and harassment; and public and private space. A wide range of recommendations are made concerning the design and maintenance of specialist and ordinary housing, as well as the local environs, points which should be considered by all those with an interest in the environment in which older people live.

Thinking about the future

Within this discussion of the special issues facing older women and their housing environments, the position of those women living alone is particularly disadvantaged: as *homeowners* they experience problems over finance, over home maintenance and repairs, over whether to 'stay put' or to move; as *tenants* some of the issues remain the same but in addition there are the problems of tackling difficult landlords on their own and dealing with increasing rents; as *residents of residential settings* they face the problem of being within the majority, but the majority that often has difficulty in finding a voice; and as *community residents* they may face all the inconveniences of an environment that does not recognize their needs. These are all issues that call for better advice for older women about housing issues; more diversity in housing types, tenures and financing; greater cooperation between agencies concerned with planning, housing, income support and social care; and a general recognition that as we age those continuities and changes we experience are reflected in our accommodation.

So what then of the future? In looking forward it is interesting to consider how the older women of future generations might differ in their needs for accommodation and community facilities. The idea of housing careers or housing biographies as a means of helping us to understand something of the diversity of experience across the life course is useful here. Such research would help us answer questions such as: 'do different generations hold different attitudes to accommodation and care in later life?'

As a starting point for this discussion the contributors to this book were asked to look at their own housing careers and those of their mother. While by no means scientific, representative or systematic, these brief housing biographies from a group of white professional women point to some interesting differences between mothers and daughters that may form a useful basis for further research. Mothers had a greater experience of rented accommodation in childhood, often moving into owner-occupied property upon marriage. Their experience of sharing accommodation was most typically with other members of their own or their partners' families. Daughters, on the other hand, had a far greater range of housing experiences at a younger age, and had more experience of sharing accommodation with non-relatives, especially as students or young workers in flats rather than houses. Daughters also had greater experience of furnished and unfurnished accommodation, and revealed greater geographical mobility, and a greater control over housing finances. Even with this most limited of exercises we are already learning something about the different experiences of living arrangements that will no doubt have a bearing on attitudes towards accommodation and care in later life. We need to know more about the influence of age, race and class on these experiences, as well as the impact of those dominant ideologies within society which shape women's patterns of accommodation.

This chapter has shown that although the primacy of the domestic role of women within our society has helped shape the environment in which we live, in many ways women have failed to exert control over this area. It is important that the housing experiences of the present generations of older women are understood by those currently in a position to advise and support women in these areas. Younger women should recognize the strengths and weaknesses of their own experiences of accommodation and the environments in which they live as they enter later life.

8 A Third Age lifestyle for older women?

Miriam Bernard and Kathy Meade

'. . . when you've worked all your life, I mean, you shouldn't have to live like a hermit. Well, we don't you see. Some people say, Oh we can save money. Well, I could if I lived like a hermit all year round. But we're in the WEA, we go to classes, we're in the Labour Party, the Antiquarian Society, And you know we support Oxfam and Save the Children, things like which you're perfectly entitled to do if you've worked all your life. Surely you're entitled to a bit of leisure.'

(Ray)

Introduction

The now prevailing image of retirement, or as it is increasingly promoted, the Third Age, is of a time of opportunity for personal development, a time of freedom, of leisure and pleasure. How meaningful, we need to ask, is this new perspective for older women? What do we know about how they use their time? How much choice do they have over how that time is spent? What are the similarities and differences between them?

Until comparatively recently, approaches to the study of leisure in later life have tended to concentrate almost exclusively on how to spend the dramatic increase in the 'free time' that marks the end of participation in paid work. All too familiar is the emphasis, highlighted in many preretirement courses, on the need to 'develop hobbies' and 'pursue interests' as a way of replacing work and filling those endless years of undifferentiated time which seem to stretch ahead. Research too has tended to be hidebound by this activity-oriented approach to the use of time in old age; a consequence we would suggest, of our male-dominated, work-oriented culture. Indeed, it is only during the latter half of the 1980s that we have seen the emergence of a number of studies which begin to counteract the invisibility of 'leisure' in (albeit younger) women's lives (Karla Henderson *et al.*, 1989). These affirm the importance of leisure as a contributor to the quality of life that is the right of all women (Rosemary Deem, 1986; Erica Wimbush and Margaret Talbot, 1988; Eileen Green *et al.*, 1990).

Our concern in this chapter is to explore the ways in which women spend their time in later life. We begin by reviewing the various theories surrounding the meaning of leisure, before going on to outline what is known about the leisure pursuits of older women. We explore the failure of research to date to focus on older women and to acknowledge their diversity. Using a feminist analysis we then examine three sets of constraints that restrict women's current, and potential, experience of leisure in later life. These are: first, the constraints imposed by the gender division of labour and women's work; second, the impact of age, both in terms of being shaped by history and by prevalent attitudes towards old age; and third, the gender-based social and economic factors which differentially affect the leisure choices of older men and women.

Defining leisure

Although many writers have grappled with the notion of leisure in relation to the quality of life, there is general agreement that we have usually considered it in terms of three broad categories:

- in connection with work
- in relation to time
- in terms of its meaning for the individual

Feminists have criticized the first two approaches for being 'gender blind' and for viewing women, if at all, as deviant cases, or solely as part of the family (Deem, 1986). We would add to this, arguing that leisure as a traditional concept has also been age-blind and has little relevance to the lives of older women.

Work—the opposite of leisure

In a society which views paid work as *the* central life interest it is not surprising that leisure has come to be seen as the opposite of this: as time for rest and recuperation (literally re-creation for more work!). Essentially, leisure became defined as non-work, significant only because of its connection with work. At the risk of over-simplification, life was seen to be readily compartmentalized between work and leisure and men were seen to earn leisure through (full-time) paid work (Wilensky, 1960; Parker, 1972; Kelly, 1972). This conceptual starting point led to a preoccupation in both theoretical and empirical writings on leisure with 'the working man' and his leisure activities (Miriam Bernard, 1982; Green *et al.*, 1990; Sue

McIntosh, 1981; Margaret Talbot, 1979). Yet, despite changes in employment patterns for both men and women, the reduction in working hours, and the lengthening of the period spent in 'retirement', this approach to leisure remains little altered. In purely quantitative terms the relation between paid work and leisure may have changed, yet the idea of work as key to personal fulfilment, to self-respect and identity, is still deeply engrained in our collective psychology (Bernard, 1990). Within such an ideological framework, both women's leisure and leisure in later life present difficulties.

Recent writings on (younger) women and leisure argue that the paid work/leisure dichotomy has rendered women's leisure invisible. Their leisure cannot simply be equated with time away from labour market activities. Where women have been considered it has been primarily in relation to their home and family responsibilities. Since, this argument runs, the primary focus of 'women's work' was the family, and since domesticity (and motherhood) were the sources of women's pleasure, then they had little need of leisure (Young and Willmott, 1973; Rapoport and Rapoport, 1975). On its own, however, 'women's work' was not perceived to earn for women the same right to leisure. Yet neither did their paid work, for it was assumed that since women in general did not participate continuously in the labour market, then leisure must play a less significant role in their lives than in men's. Thus, the sexual division of labour has had a profound effect on the leisure experiences of women.

The juxtaposition of paid work and leisure is similarly problematic for older people. Leisure without its antithesis of work is rendered meaningless; the 'free time' which is the 'reward' of retirement is consequently devalued. In essence this perspective can 'reinforce a definition of him or her (the older person) as out of date and functionless since leisure is generally viewed as superfluous in character' (Dobbin, 1980). To counter this a number of roles have been ascribed to leisure in later life—either to compensate in various ways for the loss of work roles (Brehm, 1968; de Carlo, 1974), or to help provide necessary continuity in people's lives (Atchley, 1971; Long, 1989). Indeed, one recent study (Long and Wimbush, 1985) highlights a number of different ways in which retirees (all men!) incorporate leisure activities into ways of coping with the changes brought about by retirement from paid work, although all respondents still expressed a desire to be involved in 'productive activity'. Unfortunately, this work-substitution model does not really help us understand the role of leisure in later life. As in many other comparable studies of retirement, leisure simply becomes redefined to encompass both personally and socially meaningful activity (the 'work' of later life?) and 'idle pleasure'.

For older women, it is plausible that the gender- and age-based challenges to the paid work/leisure perspective might converge in the context of retirement. Until recently, most of the literature on retirement concentrated on the experience of men. Retirement, the argument went, was of prime importance to men because it marked a fundamental status change: that from worker to non-worker, and involved a substantial period of adjustment to one's altered circumstances. Women, on the other hand, even if they had been in paid employment, would find the retirement transition easier largely because of the 'other roles' (the women's work!) they were still likely to be engaged in, and which they could readily substitute for work. Maxine Szinovacz (1982) counters this, arguing first, that there is little evidence that discontinuity in employment correlates with a lack of commitment that might make for an easier adjustment to retirement, and second, that domestic tasks are unlikely to provide an effective substitute for the personal, social and material rewards of paid employment. This line of reasoning would suggest that the concerns cited earlier about the work/leisure axis similarly affect older women and men. However, as we will discuss later, the additional gender issues surrounding women's work and leisure appear to influence women's experience of leisure throughout the life course.

Time, and leisure

Time, and particularly the notion of 'free time', has been the other principal way of defining leisure in our industrialized society. Free time is linked with notions of 'residual time' (i.e. subtracting anything not regarded as leisure such as sleep and other basic needs); with 'discretionary time' (implying choice about how to use that time); and to ideas about 'filling time'. However, as with work-related definitions, time on its own does not appear to offer a very useful conceptualization for women (Betsy Wearing and Stephen Wearing, 1988). In the first place, time-bound definitions suggest that we can divide up our time into easily recognized and delimited parts, which is patently not the case for many women, especially if they are not in paid employment outside the home. For example, the leisure component in preparing a special meal for friends contrasts markedly with everyday cooking. Conversely, what may be commonly perceived as leisure activities can also be regarded as work, e.g. gardening, voluntary work, attending sewing classes. Even where women can separate work from leisure, the time available for them to pursue activities or interests of their own choice is often fragmented (Deem, 1986). Second, research has shown that some groups of women feel they do not deserve, or have the time, to engage in leisure activities (Bernard, 1983; Wearing and Wearing, 1988). A pervasive ethic of care, which socializes women into placing the needs of others before her own, prompts feelings of guilt if she allows herself to 'indulge' in leisure

(Carol Gilligan, 1982; Ann Oakley, 1984). Third, even if there is time available (and other resources such as money and transport), several writers have argued that gender role expectations will rule how it is spent. The social construct of 'femininity' and of 'appropriate behaviour' place limitations on women—the disapproval shown towards women on their own in pubs, or those going out without their partners are but two examples (Deem, 1986; Green *et al.*, 1990).

Despite this, 'time' seems to be an enduring quality in relation to definitions of leisure. But, as Karla Henderson (1990) contends, 'the concept of time has limited applicability unless it is considered within other contexts of women's lives' (p.231). For older women it is evident that issues concerning time and leisure, as with work and leisure, come together in the context of retirement. With the lowering of retirement age and increases in longevity, we are likely to be spending as much time 'in retirement' as 'in work' in the late twentieth century. Retirement, it is now argued, is a distinct part of the life course, replete with additional free time (Long and Wimbush, 1979; Laslett, 1989; Lazcko and Phillipson, 1991). In this postcareer, postchild-rearing phase of life, it might be reasonable to assume that the gender-based constraints on women's leisure time would disappear. Age, we contend later however, does not prove to be a great leveller.

The leisure experience

In the light of dissatisfaction with these traditional conceptualizations around time, work and activity, some recent studies of women and leisure, and to a lesser extent studies of later life, have begun to concentrate on the meaning of the experience of leisure. The thrust of this approach has been based on the premise that work and leisure should no longer be:

> 'regarded as separate spheres but instead as a complex set of experiences involving degrees of freedom and constraint. When the "grey" areas between work and play become a major focus of research instead of being tacked on as an afterthought to the main model, it becomes easier to site leisure in context' (Green *et al.*, 1990, p.19).

It is the quality of the experience that makes the activity leisure, not the activity itself (Henderson *et al.*, 1989). What is important is how the individual feels. There is no single meaning for leisure: free choice, relaxation, sociability, creativity, self-expression, enjoyment and escape from the obligations of social roles, have all been described as elements of a meaningful leisure experience (Green *et al.*, 1990; Kelly, 1990). The form of the leisure experience may be equally varied: demanding, social or solitary, intense or relaxing, regular or occasional. Indeed, the same activity may have different meanings at different times in the life course. Implicit is the positive contribution leisure experiences can make to the quality of life, and life satisfaction. From this perspective, leisure is not: 'a left over or segmented element of life. Rather it is integrated with the meanings, aims, relationships, identities and constraints that run through the other domains of life such as family, community and work' (Kelly, 1990, p.154).

This conception is perhaps the most useful way of understanding this aspect of women's lives because it enables us to look in a holistic way at how women's roles intermesh without artificially focusing on specific issues such as use of time or activity (Rachel Dixey, 1987). Moreover, in challenging the work-derivation model of leisure, and stressing the context of the multiple roles that change and intersect over the life course, this approach is, we believe, equally helpful for exploring leisure experiences in later life.

The lifestyles of older women

Engagement in leisure has been identified as a crucial dimension of wellbeing in later life (Havighurst, 1963; Kelly, 1990; Bernard, 1985). Certainly regular participation in social and other activities outside the home, has consistently correlated with higher levels of life satisfaction among older adults (Kelly, 1990). Several explanations for this finding have been offered: leisure activity provides continuity of valued non-work roles, a context for social interaction, and opportunity for satisfying personal expression and development (Kelly, 1990; Thompson *et al.*, 1990).

We turn now to look more closely at the lifestyles of older women: to explore the meaning of leisure in their lives and its impact on their quality of life. This discussion looks critically at what we know about how older women spend their time, at how far the constraints surrounding 'free time' continue across the life course, and at whether gender relations and the sexual division of labour continue to influence the experience of leisure. We are mindful of the limitations to this discussion: there have been few empirical or longitudinal studies in the UK that have sought to understand the leisure experience of older women. Our material is pieced together from what exists— some large-scale surveys and a few small-scale biographical studies. Our arguments are exploratory.

Resourcefulness

Before we begin, it is imperative to stress the resourcefulness many older women exhibit and the rich patterns of their lives. Without acknowledging and describing some of this richness, there is a danger of developing what could appear to be a negative, deficit model of women's lives in old age. For, despite being multiply and objectively disadvantaged in many ways, the leisure patterns and lifestyles of older women in fact reveal remarkable variation (Parker, 1985; Deem, 1986; Janet Ford and Ruth Sinclair, 1987).

The enterprise of some older married women in carving out time and space for themselves is clearly shown in Jennifer Mason's work (1987a). One woman for example, likes 'mooching' around the shops on her own, but in order to be able to do so, she deliberately waits until her husband is up the top of a ladder before getting her bag and coat, shouting, 'bye dear' and disappearing off out quickly before he can get down and accompany her. Other women in Mason's study manage to achieve the same ends by different means: either through a process of negotiation, by default or by conflict.

The ability of some women to counter constraints such as decreased mobility, language and cultural differences, limited networks, low income, and environmental barriers is also evident. An empirical study of Leisure Provision and People's Need (Dower *et al.*, 1979), features elderly women living alone. The authors describe Mrs Holly aged 82 who, despite her poor state of health, her relative immobility and her lack of financial resources:

> 'has the ability to attract people and to make friendships . . . has a keen sense of humour . . . and is an optimistic person and takes things in her own time: she manages to conserve her energy so that she can do the things she wants. She has started to attend a social group once a week, go to church, and to make regular visits to a hairdresser. She derives companionship as well as service support from her home help, and looks forward to going to stay with her grand-daughter out of London when invited and fetched' (para 8.126).

Mrs Gandhi, one of the women interviewed by Janet Ford and Ruth Sinclair (1987) similarly works hard to construct a satisfactory life:

> 'Every day I go into town and buy some food and come back and cook. I enjoy that very much because I can choose for myself and because I am learning I want to learn more. I want to learn to speak English and maybe learn to read or write. Two people from the church have started to teach me to speak English. My husband (who she left a year ago) did not think it was important for me to learn and he would not let me . . .' (p.43).

In discussing their in-depth interviews with older women, Ford and Sinclair confirm the findings of research with younger women:

> '. . . what is also apparent is that the relationship between the various needs in their lives is a complex one. Status, self-respect and interest come from interacting with others in a way that conveys a sense of value and enjoyment. These activities also give a sense of personal control and choice . . .' (p.152).

Most importantly these life stories illustrate how older women actively pursue creating a satisfying life for themselves. For each older woman there is evidence of a dynamic and creative tension between constraint and opportunity.

Older women and leisure activities

It has been argued earlier that the activity checklist approach which has been used in leisure research has not captured the contextual complexity surrounding some leisure (or work) activities. Nevertheless, an analysis of older women's participation in 'leisure activities' is still of considerable use, even if only to highlight the shortcomings of the research methodologies.

The early large-scale leisure surveys (Rodgers, 1967; Sillitoe, 1969) revealed an aggregate pattern of declining participation with increasing age. This has been borne out in later social surveys such as the 1986 GHS (OPCS, 1989a; CSO, 1989; 1990). On the whole, participation declines both for indoor and outdoor pursuits, although some notable exceptions to this trend are levels of participation in bowling and gardening. Other activities remain at fairly consistent levels over the life course, declining, if at all, only when we reach the 70 and over age groups. These predominantly home-based and domestic activities include watching television, visiting or entertaining friends or relations, reading books, dressmaking, needlework and knitting. With physical activities and sport, the highest level of participation is the 5 per cent of women aged 60 and over who now take part in keep-fit activities such as yoga and aerobics. This is followed by 3 per cent who swim; 2 per cent who cycle; and only 1 per cent who play golf, bowls or darts. As Eric Midwinter has recently observed in his report to the Carnegie Enquiry (1992):

> 'Bearing in mind the approximate sex ratio in late age of 2 to 1 in favour of women, it may be estimated that relatively few women are involved in these recreations. A rough assessment might suggest that, out of the eight million of females of pensionable age, only about three-quarters of a million take part in any outdoor exercise' (p.7).

We also have some statistical information about participation in educational and voluntary activities. Three national surveys conducted in the early 1980s indicated that between 3 per cent and 9 per cent of people over 65 attended 'leisure classes' or courses (OPCS, 1983b; 1985; Advisory Council for Adult and Continuing Education, 1982). These surveys also tell us that older women are twice as likely as older men to participate in adult education. A recent study by Naomi Sargant (1991) suggests that participation has increased, with 9 per cent of people over 65 undertaking some form of formal study and another 6 per cent engaged in informal learning through community groups and clubs. Moreover, additional analysis indicates that there no longer appears to be a significant difference in participation between older men and women in formal study. Indeed, if anything, older men over 50 have become more involved than older women in learning and studying (18 per cent as opposed to 13 per cent, respectively). The involvement of older people in voluntary work is higher and shows only a small difference between older women and men. The 1987 GHS indicates that 14 per cent of women over 70 years (13 per cent of men) and 25 per cent of women aged 60–69 (19 per cent of men) were engaged in some form of voluntary activity during the preceding year (Jil Matheson, 1990). While similar proportions of volunteers of all age groups were involved in fundraising and serving on committees (approximately 40 per cent), older volunteers were more likely to be giving practical help to people such as providing transport, domestic help or gardening, and visiting people in hospitals or residential homes.

From other studies we know, for example, that approximately 30 per cent of older women join social clubs but only 13 per cent attend clubs that cater solely for older people and about 11 per cent go to bingo. More are involved in religious-based activities (Abrams, 1978; 1980; Dorothy Jerrome, 1990a; Thompson *et al.*, 1990). This finding also applies to older people from black and minority ethnic groups. A survey in Nottingham revealed that churchgoing was the most common social activity amongst West Indian pensioners, with 74 per cent of older women attending weekly compared with 46 per cent of older men (Berry *et al.*, 1981). Similar findings have been reported from other communities, including Jewish pensioners in South London (Jimack, 1983), Afro-Caribbean and Asian elders in Birmingham (Bhalla and Blakemore, 1981) and in Coventry (Bruce Holland and Gillian Levando-Hundt, 1987), and elderly people from the New Commonwealth and Pakistan in Derby (Lambert and Dolan, 1986).

Visiting and being visited is another common form of leisure activity and social contact. The 1985 GHS (OPCS, 1987a) reveals that outgoing visits decrease with age—65 per cent of women aged 65–69 visit friends and relatives once a week or more compared with only 24 per cent of women aged 85 or over. The figures for incoming visits remain more constant, with about two-thirds of older people receiving one or more visitors each week. Conversely, about one-fifth of older people rarely visit friends or relatives and one-quarter are rarely visited. We are talking here of nearly two million people who see close contacts only once a month or even less.

Holiday-taking is a popular index of the leisure lifestyle of older people, but in reality older people are less likely to take a holiday than most of the adult population. In 1985 47 per cent of retired people spent four nights or more away from home compared with 58 per cent of the total population (OPCS, 1987a). Older people also holiday abroad at half of the rate of other adults. There is also a marked decline in holiday-making as people age. While 56 per cent of 65 to 70-year-olds took holidays in 1985, only 28 per cent of people over 80 did so.

Overall, it must be said that these surveys paint a somewhat gloomy portrait of later life. Given the increase in people's free time after ceasing paid work, we might have expected to see evidence of a greater involvement in a wide range of social, educational and physical activities. This is not the case. Most of the available data suggest that older people are engaged in more passive activity for a significant proportion of each day. An examination of television viewing is illustrative: in 1988 people over 65 watched, on average, 37 hours 25 minutes per week (OPCS, 1990a).

Limitations of current research *Age/ Gender.*

Revealing though such participation surveys are, they do have a number of severe limitations when considering later life in general and older women in particular.

First, there are problems in the way they deal with age itself. For example, some early leisure surveys either excluded elderly people altogether or considered them as one homogeneous group over a certain age (Sillitoe, 1969). Later surveys, such as those from Age Concern England (Abrams, 1978; 1980) did at least begin to acknowledge the heterogeneity in a 'group' whose ages might span 30 or 40 years, by subdividing the older age groups into two or more categories. Even so, greater differentiation by age will only provide a rough correlation with increasing frailty and accompanying restrictions on some kinds of activity. Comparing information across surveys has also proved difficult because of the inconsistent age divisions that are employed. The 1981 GHS (OPCS, 1983b) on voluntary activity for example, uses 65–74 and 75 plus age bands, whereas that in 1987 (OPCS, 1989a) groups people in 60–69 and 70 plus categories!

A second area of difficulty concerns gender. Sometimes survey results are not gender-differentiated, or are not differentiated equally across all age groups. In Sillitoe's (1969) study for example, all the age groups under 61 years are subdivided by what he terms 'domestic age' (i.e. by marital status and the presence/absence of children). However, older women are subdivided into two groups on the basis of marital status alone, i.e. 'married' and 'widowed, etc.', whilst older men are subdivided according to employment status, i.e. 'in full-time employment' or 'retired'! This sends a clear message about the relation of older men with leisure compared with older women: for the men, work is the crucial differentiating factor; for the women it is marital status. Here again, cross-comparisons are rendered difficult because of the inconsistencies in the treatment of gender in different studies.

Third, our understanding (and any action we might take) would be furthered not only by looking at the differences between men and women, but by also examining the similarities and differences between groups of older women. For example, we know that older women's participation in adult education is greater than men's. The Advisory Council for Adult and Continuing Education (1982) found that older adults who left school at 17 or over were three times more likely to attend classes, and that while 75 per cent of the older adults in the survey population came from semi- and unskilled working-class backgrounds, this was so for only 20 per cent of the older students (McNair, 1984). In this instance, class is shown to be a significant factor alongside gender in influencing who does what. The use of class to differentiate between groups of older people is often problematic for, as with gender, the defining factors differ from study to study (see p.12).

Fourth, we are also very conscious of the real lack of information about women from black and minority ethnic groups. Until recently no data on people's ethnic background had been collected systematically. However, a considerable number of small-scale studies have been undertaken in different parts of the country. These have rarely been analysed by gender, and have all too often emphasized cultural aspects as the major influence on the lifestyles of minority older people (Bhalla and Blakemore, 1981; Berry *et al.*, 1981; Barker, 1984b; Fenton, 1988; Lambert and Dolan, 1986).

Finally, there are real problems regarding the actual concepts that the surveys are trying to measure. For example, education is often measured only in terms of formal educational activity, but such figures could distort the participation levels of older adults. They may not attend classes or courses, but may well engage in learning activity through voluntary work or special interest groups (Percy, 1990; Sargant, 1991). The activity categories are also often employed on a face value basis, telling nothing of the amount of time, frequency or nature of involvement. Dancing for example, includes learning and practice, competition, physical conditioning, a round of the floor to earn afternoon tea, and/or an opportunity to socialize. Equally problematic is the notion of 'activity' itself. It carries with it connotations of being worthwhile and of being desirable. Popular but passive activities such as watching television or reading magazines carry the opposite meaning. They are labelled as time-fillers—ways of whiling away the hours. Bingo and chatting over a cup of tea (or a pint) are similarly afflicted. For older people in general, and older women in particular, this active–passive duality serves to reinforce many of the negative and damning attitudes and stereotypes we hold. Pitting activity against passivity, as much of the literature and research does, fails *pamile activ — writing, reading — Philosophy.*

to acknowledge the necessity of juxtaposing these two situations, or 'ways of being', at different times and in different proportions. Moreover, it is this kind of simplistic conceptualization of leisure that, we would suggest, is the real problem in understanding the leisure experience of older women, rather than the women themselves!—a problem they share with younger women.

Influences on the lifestyles of older women

A number of researchers have identified various sets of influences that they assert might deter or facilitate older people's ability to shape a Third Age lifestyle of their choice. The Rapoports (1975) for example, highlight education, income and health. Peterson (1983) described potential barriers under three headings: situational (e.g. lack of money or transport); dispositional (e.g. internalized negative attitudes towards old age); and institutional (e.g. inaccessible buildings or inconvenient timetabling). While these, and other typologies, might be helpful (Bernard, 1984), they are ultimately insufficient, for they fail to fully address gender relations. As Erica Wimbush and Margaret Talbot (1988) argue: 'there is a need to analyse the relational aspects of gender inequality in terms of both women's perceptions of and reactions to leisure provision, and of the underlying ideologies of the provisions made for different social groups' (p.128).

We now turn our attention to the issues that we feel are crucial to an adequate understanding of the lifestyles of older women. We aim to assess the factors that have shaped the choices older women make about how to use time and space in their lives. In the words of Jennifer Mason (1988b): 'This means analysing changing frameworks of constraint and opportunity which make possible certain patterns of leisure . . .' (p.76).

Older women and women's work

With the removal of paid work from the scenario of later life we might assume that women's and men's access to leisure time might converge. It would seem not. Recent estimates of the availability of leisure time suggest that, of the 105 waking hours per week generally available to us, a full-time employed female might expect 31 hours of 'free time', and a full time employed male, 48 hours. A retired man would have the most with 92 hours a week, while a retired woman would have 75 hours (CSO, 1990). Throughout the life course it appears that women remain more occupied with what are termed 'essential activities': domestic work, shopping, cooking, washing and so on.

These domestic and family obligations have been explored by Jennifer Mason (1987a) in her research into long term marriage. Her study of eighteen couples, all aged between 50 and 70, begins to tease out some of the ways in which leisure features in the construction of married life. Her findings bear out the Rapoports' (1975) much earlier contention that:

> 'For different sub populations strategies for relating home and family activities to work and other interests vary. The bald reporting of the fact that most 'free time' is spent in home-centred activities (as is done in most surveys) can hide the problem of just how much this is, when it is, what it consists of and how different family members work out their separate as well as their joint interests at home' (p.254).

Mason reveals that this 'working out' of interests between husbands and wives is especially important in later life. She shows that older couples have indeed begun to focus their attentions and their time much more on the home, 'and that this in many ways represented an encroachment by men on what had formerly been viewed (often by default) as women's domain, or territory' (Mason, 1988a, p.34). Although most of the women in her sample had in fact worked outside the home, they had spent more time in it than their husbands, had been in control of domestic and household routines and, as a result, had been able to exert a degree of autonomy over the use of time and space within the home (Mason, 1988b). Moreover, not only did husbands encroach on wives' personal time and space, but as Mason goes on to indicate, their presence was beginning to create different forms of domestic work for their wives (such as cooking a proper lunch where they would previously have had a snack). The women were also placed under additional pressure in terms of facilitating and supporting their husbands' new-found leisure in retirement, even to the extent of modifying their own activities. Long-term marriages are thus not without their conflicts, (see p.92), and for older women in this situation, it may in fact be exceedingly difficult to carve out leisure for themselves.

In contrast, the widows interviewed by Thompson *et al.* (1990) conveyed a 'powerful sense of fulfilment in the discovery of previously stifled independence and energy' (p.225). All saw themselves as much better off now than if they were to be locked in marriage again. As one Verity Hampshire saw it:

> 'Since I've been a widow, I'm more active. Because I have to get out and do things now, you see there's nobody else. I'm not tied down to the house either. So I find that it's good to get out . . . I found that was the best thing I could've done—to go into the community and get involved' (p.226).

Relationships with husbands then are but one aspect, for we must also acknowledge that women in later life may also be involved in other kinds of partnerships, family care and domestic labour that will influence their leisure opportunities. Some may have adult children still living at home, either because they have not left or because they have returned, following divorce for example. Other women may have considerable caring responsibilities for elderly and/or sick relatives, while yet others may be heavily involved in the care of grandchildren. Consequently, later life may not automatically herald a future of uninterrupted or autonomous leisure time for older women.

As discussed earlier there is a duality about women's work which means that while family and domestic life may have its constraints it also caters for their leisure needs. This too continues into later life. Consider the case of Mrs C for example. She is a 75-year-old resident of a small village near Newhaven in East Sussex whose life has been dominated by the domestic routine and the demands of building up a dairy business with her husband (Tomlinson, 1979). Concerning leisure, she observes that: 'We didn't know we was missing anything. It was work, work, work and we didn't know no better. We had no time for leisure. It was all routine then.'

This routine, involving work, family and domestic commitments, was a coherent whole in which her leisure needs were, and still are, satisfied through home and family-centred activities, plus some outside involvements such as with the Women's Institute. As she herself says: 'I've always done three things marvellously, . . . knitting, gardening and talking', and it is around these that her leisure has been constructed. She recalls that on Thursdays, the women of the village sewed together in one or other of their houses, whilst a more spontaneous and improvised social activity might be the day-long blackberrying or raspberrying trips, on which thirty or more mothers and children would go.

Mrs C's biography highlights the marked gender division of labour; the lack of any clear dividing line between work and leisure, and the importance of a social life constructed around domestic activities carried out largely in the company of other women. In later life this pattern seems to be strengthened if anything. At this point, the demographic imperative coincides most forcefully with women's greater tendency to form and maintain friendships with other women. Sociability continues to be a particularly strong theme in the satisfaction that older women, like younger women, derive from their leisure (Parker, 1985; Green *et al.*, 1990). Furthermore, much of this continues to be set in the context of shared leisure activity with other women around 'women's work': informal family and social visiting, voluntary work, shopping trips, and involvement in church groups (Jerrome, 1990a).

Cohort analysis

Not at your age . . . generation and gender

There has been some debate about the cohort effect for the current
generation of older people and their participation in certain types of
leisure, especially 'active' sports, recreational and educational activities outside the home (Rapoport and Rapoport, 1975; Groombridge,
1980, Shea, 1990). History-related influences, it is argued, have negatively affected their leisure expectations. People born in the 1920s and
1930s were strongly influenced by the Depression and the stigma linked
to unemployment. The postwar period reinforced the work ethic,
emphasizing the value of work and the problems arising from 'too
much leisure' (Johnston and Phillipson, 1983). This generation was
also denied access to education, yet at the same time their experience
of it often held a 'sweet/sour taste' (Groombridge, 1980). They also
grew up in an era in which public provision for leisure and recreation
was comparatively minimal. These factors meant that few people ever
included formal recreational or educational activities as a regular part
of their life beyond school, making it difficult to take them up, out of
character as it were, in later life. Very many of this cohort of older people
will never have visited a leisure centre or adult education institute, believing such facilities as 'not for the likes of us'. In theory this cohort of older
people may be well placed to take advantage of recreational, cultural and
educational facilities; in reality they generally fail to do so.

The theory of generation, and the power of shared experience
across the life course can be challenged for failing to account for the
enormous diversity among older people. It can also be criticized for
the rather fatalistic picture it presents. Nevertheless, there is value
in an historical analysis that acknowledges the gender dimension
along with class and race. Let us consider then, as a brief illustration,
the educational background of today's older women and its impact
on leisure activity.

Among the present population aged 65 and over, some 70 per cent
left school at the age of 13 or 14 and only 5 per cent of the men, and
3 per cent of the women went on to further or higher education. In
addition to the general lack of educational opportunity, this cohort
of women suffered from deep-seated and largely negative social attitudes towards the education of women. One woman's story mirrors
the experience of many others, surveyed in this instance by the European Older Students Research Group:

> 'My mother said in 1933, you can't go to High School, I don't believe in
> education for GIRLS; she kept on having babies and only my two younger
> brothers went to High School owing to the 1944 Education Act. One is
> an architect and one an insurance manager . . . my sisters never went to
> high school either . . . if we had been born in a later age I am sure every
> single one of us would have gone to College' (Stephanie Clennell, 1990,
> p.64).

Useful knowledge for women was usually defined as that of domestic value. Women's educational experience (or dearth of it) was designed primarily to prepare them for their roles as wives and mothers. Women's talents and capabilities were largely suppressed in the interests of the gender division of labour. This, feminists contend, reinforced male superiority and left many women with feelings of inadequacy and a lack of confidence that limited their horizons to home, family and largely unskilled work (Jane Thompson, 1983). While the particular woman above went on to rectify her lack of opportunity through an Open University course when she retired, she is the exception rather than the rule. The vast majority, 'the missing millions of working class people' as they have been described, have never entered another educational establishment, either for vocational, liberal or hobby-type classes (Jill Liddington, 1986).

It should come as no surprise to find that the small percentage of mainly middle-class older women who do participate are to be found in adult education centres where there is still by and large 'a women's curriculum' of craft and homemaking, and that there are certain subject areas where older women rarely feature, such as carpentry and technology.

The type of informal education women received could also influence their leisure pursuits. Talbot (1979) argues that women are less trained in the skills necessary for many sorts of leisure activity and contends that:

> 'Their mothers, schools or peers pass on to them "domestic" skills like knitting and sewing, but the socialization process tends to miss out gross motor skills, handicrafts in wood and metal, informal pub games and driving. The ability to take part in many forms of recreation depends to a large extent on the "qualifications" of skills of this type and this appears to be one constraint which precludes women's participation in both institutionalized and informal recreation' (p.32).

If access to these skills was denied to women in their younger years, it was probable that women's participation was likely to be circumscribed throughout their entire life course. Swimming, ball games and do-it-yourself activities spring most immediately to mind.

It is not a major step from the debate about generation and gender, to constructions of 'age and gender-appropriate' leisure activities. The image of leisure is youthful, fit, active and largely male, if media coverage or usage of sports facilities or leisure centres is any guide (Veal, 1981). This popular image reflects particular representations of gender and age as well as race, class and disability. Analyses of gender representation highlight the use of women's sexuality to promote leisure (e.g. in alcohol, travel or exercise bike advertisements). Youth and beauty predominate, rendering ageing women invisible unless they are Jane Fondas, or part of the new stylishly ageing JOLLIES (jet-setting oldies with lots of loot) or WOOPIES (well-off older people) who, as the acronyms suggest, have the financial resources for leisure pursuits. In such a youth-oriented society both middle-aged and older women struggle with ageism as well as sexism. The ideology is a powerful sanction on how women may choose to spend their leisure time. Women are forced into increasing self-consciousness about their bodies as they age. This makes going swimming difficult, for instance, as well as many other forms of physical activity (Vera Ivers, 1984). Preconceptions that falsely equate old age with ill health (see p.70) may further restrict the range of physical recreation activities on offer to, or readily taken up by, older women.

Other stereotypes that diminish the capabilities of older people, e.g. inability to learn new things, have a further impact. Early cross-sectional studies compared the 'intelligence', and especially the memory capacity of younger people with older people and found older people wanting. Although these studies have largely been discredited, ageist perceptions of capability nevertheless continue to influence the range of opportunities available to older people (Shea, 1990). At its least subtle, this can be seen in the age discrimination that stops older people from being active in, for example, the Girl Guide movement from 65, holding office in the Women's Royal Voluntary Service at 65 or being a member of a Community Health Council at 70 (Midwinter, 1990).

Challenging the myth that 'you can't teach an old dog new tricks' by taking up new pursuits requiring new knowledge and skills, requires considerable self-confidence. Some experimental studies with younger people show that in instances where men and women have equal ability and are equally keen to succeed, men are much more confident than women (Nicholson, 1984). Given the influences of generation outlined above, we would infer that a similar gender difference might exist within older age groups. These factors may well contribute to the findings of the Older Student Group (Clennell, 1987) at the Open University, which indicate that older women are much less likely than older men to tackle award-bearing courses.

Such perceptions, and particularly negative self-perceptions, can accentuate the constraints linked to historical and ideological forces. Older women's leisure choices, like those of everyone else, are made from within that 'relatively narrow range which at the time are compatible with their way of life and above all, their perception of themselves' (Mills, 1976).

Gender inequality: out and about

While all the literature demonstrates that women's leisure is more home-based than that of men, it is certainly a matter for debate that this is women's choice. Alongside continuing gender-based norms of acceptable leisure activity, personal fear of male violence on the street and the lack of adequate public transport are powerful constraints on (older) women's use of free time. Resource factors, both in terms of income and material goods, are also highly influential.

A major study by Mark Abrams (1980) of people over 75, two-thirds of whom were women, indicated that home-based leisure activities took up most of their free time. Only one-third of the respondents had been out on the day before the interview. Bhalla and Blakemore's Birmingham survey (1981) corroborates this, showing that trips out of the house appear to be much less common for Asian, Afro-Caribbean and European older women than for older men. While over 80 per cent of their sample of Asian and European men leave the house daily, only 35 per cent of Asian women and 60 per cent of European women do so. For women, these figures challenge the commonly held stereotype of the 'housewife' who continues to pop out to do her daily shopping. Indeed there is also some research evidence to show that this stereotype does not even hold for younger women and that there is a strong unmet need just to be able to get out of the house (Bernard, 1983).

A later study undertaken by the former Greater London Council Women's Committee (1985) also shows the impact of age and gender on travel patterns. Over three-quarters of the women over 75 years did some walking each week, but they were much less likely to use other forms of transport such as private cars, British Rail, the Underground or taxis. Shopping was their main purpose for going out, but 40 per cent of their journeys were 'for pleasure': a lower frequency than for younger women.

As we discussed earlier in the context of marriage and women's work, a woman may need considerable skill and confidence to assert her right to independent leisure outside the home. Traditional female activities which coincide with the role of wife and mother appear to meet with comparatively little resistance from partners, so long as they do not interfere with domestic responsibilities. Keep fit, flower arranging, or church activities are such examples. Other activities such as nights out unaccompanied by male partners, or escorts, are certainly perceived as less acceptable for younger women and are cause for conflict (Deem, 1986; Green *et al.*, 1990). Concepts of socially acceptable and respectable activity, based on constructs of female sexuality, continue to hold considerable sway. In the absence of research we would assume this to be true in the same way for older women. Elderly men seeking company have the choice to go to the pub or working men's club, but this is still not a viable option for lone or lonely older women. It is therefore no surprise that the bingo hall, which has traditionally been a woman's domain and hence perceived as a suitably safe environment, attracts considerable numbers of older working-class women (Dixey and Talbot, 1982).

Rosemary Deem (1986) argues that women's leisure outside the home is often 'policed' by the actions of men and their control of public spaces. It manifests itself in women's well-founded fear of male violence and their consequent curtailing of activity. In the Greater London Council Women's Committee study cited above, mobility problems were shown to prevent women, and particularly those over 75, from going out, but an even more major constraint on women's travel patterns was identified—fear for their personal safety. While common to a significant proportion of women of all ages (30 per cent), well over half of the women over 60 identified strong anxieties about using public transport as well as walking out after dark. In the words of the report: 'It is very clear that a very high proportion of elderly and Asian women in particular are severely restricted in their activities at night by fear of attack and have adjusted their lives in order to avoid the need to go out alone' (p.8). Indeed, 70 per cent reported never going out on their own after dark. Even in the daytime only one-third felt safe using British Rail or the Underground, and two-thirds felt safe walking. In other large cities similar findings would be likely, and in rural areas public transport is noted for its infrequency and unreliability.

Access to safe transport is clearly key. A whole range of leisure and educational pursuits are facilitated by car ownership. However, people of pensionable age are twice as likely not to have access to a car as other adults. Women bear the brunt of this disadvantage, for even if they reside in a household which possesses a vehicle it is unlikely that they themselves will hold a driving licence. In Mason's study (1988a), only two women, compared with 17 men, were able to drive and had personal access to a car. In households with a car and in which the woman can drive, it may not necessarily be available to them, especially if the woman is retired and her husband still works.

Older people's lack of access to private transport and their reliance on public transport is indicative of their income status. An acute lack of income is possibly the most limiting constraint on the leisure activities of older people. An impoverished financial picture led Maggie Pearson (1991) to conclude that among black and minority ethnic older people who are either in or approaching retirement, 'their new found leisure may be bleak, with very few real choices' (p.440). Moreover, as Dulcie Groves has shown in Chapter 3, older women are, in particular, greatly disadvantaged in financial terms; a situation which often reflects a lifetime of unequal opportunity for either earning their own, or gaining access to, an adequate income. The costs of leisure and recreational equipment, entrance fees to classes, swimming pools, museums or theatre tickets and so on, can be well beyond the reach of many older women, further confining her to less-expensive leisure activities indoors.

These financial constraints do not bear equally on all sectors of the older population. There are some relatively affluent older households that include women. But, as Mason's (1987b) work shows, simply quantifying a household's gross income says nothing about who controls or manages the money. Indeed, while most of her couples talked about the need to tighten their financial belts in retirement, it was evident that even in the more affluent households, husbands were the ones who exerted the most control over how that income was spent. For older women who do not have access to their own money, the fact of always having to ask for money to pursue leisure activities can call the legitimacy of that activity into question (Mason, 1988b). Furthermore, if as Peter Laslett (1989) contends, the control of economic resources has been, and still is, in the hands of males, how can women ever hope to be in a position to live a Third Age lifestyle?

Shaping a Third Age lifestyle for older women

In this chapter we have sought to outline the current state of knowledge about the leisure lives of older women. We have argued that leisure can only be adequately understood within a framework that takes account of the totality of women's lives, and which acknowledges that this is structured by a variety of complex, and gender-related, influences.

We have had two critical obstacles to contend with. First, British women-centred research around leisure has almost completely neglected older women. Second, British gerontologists have failed by and large to address leisure, despite the fact that the significance of leisure activity in later life is not a new issue (Kelly, 1990). This has meant that while we have been able to support the feminist challenge to the inadequacy of traditional conceptualizations of leisure and extend it theoretically to include older women, it has proved difficult to back this with research findings. In particular, older women's perceptions of the experience of leisure have yet to be rigorously explored. We know something about how they spend their time, but little about their motivation and how they feel about what they do. Leisure has been an invisible dimension of older women's lives and, we suspect, rarely perceived as a right.

What stands out from our exploration is the continuity of gender-related influences across the life course. In the three major areas we have probed—women's work and leisure; the concept of generation and age-appropriate activity; and constraints on women's leisure outside the home—we would contend that age has not diluted the impact of gender. Tackling this gender inequality necessitates enhancing the opportunities for older women to experience the elements which leisure embodies; be it free choice, relaxation, creativity, enjoyment or social contact. Getting more older women into leisure by improving their access to existing leisure facilities and activities is, we would argue, only part of the answer. Changing older women's social and economic position is a necessary prerequisite for a better leisure environment. Only then will older women, like younger women, really have leisure of their own.

9 Women come of age

Miriam Bernard, Kathy Meade and
Anthea Tinker

'. . . it's a certain amount of achievement if you're surviving by your own efforts—at any age. I don't know what I'd feel if people said, "Oh, you mustn't do that you're getting so old" . . . What would I be like if I was in a position that I had to do what I was told by somebody? I wouldn't like that again either! I'm enjoying this bit of it really, being able to do anything, like change the garden . . . There are all sorts of things one has to try and cope with—bringing up children, divorce, moving house, living alone—and I think once you have . . . I feel I've got to a state at this moment that that sort of thing is behind me. I mean it may not be at all. But overcoming situations and eventually reaching a state of contentment of some sort . . . Some of my friends, they cope very well with what they've got to do, or the sort of lives they've got, and some don't. They just sort of sit down and crumble . . . Once they've stopped being needed . . .'

(Joan)

Introduction

Throughout this book we have striven to give voice to the key themes raised in Joanna Bornat's conversations with Ray, Joan, Pat, Charanjit and Olga (Chapter 2). Each life story gives us insight into what each woman uniquely brings to her old age, yet at the same time they collectively reflect common patterns in women's lives. We have been continually mindful of this 'tension' between acknowledging women's individual experiences, their diversity and differences, and interpolating those experiences which they share, as women.

Older women are skilful survivors, working hard to construct for themselves lives which are enjoyable and satisfying in the face of considerable constraints. At a fundamental level, older women (and men) struggle with the powerful stereotyping of old people as redundant and roleless, in a society preoccupied with chronological age and productivity. Women's visible productive role disappears as they

leave employment and, additionally for many women, when their
role in reproduction ends, and when children move away from home
and partners die. If judged against the values of such a society older
women's lives will, in the words of Janet Ford and Ruth Sinclair,
'frequently appear diminished, or even failures' (1987, p.6). It is in
this context that older people have been constructed as a 'social
problem'. For older women this pervasive ageism is compounded by
the effects of gender inequality over the life course. This is most
clearly manifested in their poverty, their lack of power and 'dependent' status.

Yet, conversely, we see vast numbers of older women who, even
when frail, are far from ground under, and who every day draw
strength from a wealth of life experience. Like the women Joanna
Bornat talked with, those interviewed by Susan Hemmings (1985),
Ford and Sinclair (1987), Suzanne Nield and Rosalind Pearson (1992)
share with us their resilience, their creativity and inventiveness, their
courage and ability to manage radical changes in their lives. Most
particularly, women counter their relative social and economic
powerlessness by actively fostering their interpersonal ties within
family networks and friendships.

The previous chapters represent an attempt to document what we
know about the position of older women, their strengths and
resources, the problems and barriers they face. In this chapter we aim
to draw those threads together. First, we explore three key themes in
older women's lives: continuity and change; dependence, independence and interdependence; and diversity and difference. These
themes, in turn, inform the subsequent discussion of an agenda for
change. The final section considers strategies for achieving these
objectives.

Key themes in older women's lives

Continuity and change

We have argued that in order to understand the lives of older women
it is necessary to adopt a life-course perspective and to look back at
what has gone before. It is folly to take a segment of a woman's life
and examine it with no appreciation of the potentially profound effect
of previous events. For example, a woman whose childhood was
spent in poverty, who left school at 15, went to work in an unskilled
job, had children and then spent years in part-time jobs, is unlikely
to have built up her own financial resources in terms of entitlement
to an earnings related pension or savings. However, she may if she
has held the strings of the family purse, have a great deal more

practical knowledge and life skills than a middle-class woman whose husband controlled the family finances.

As we learned in Chapter 2, many women experience anything but straightforward 'career' paths. Full-time work is often followed by a withdrawal from the labour market while children are born and raised. Part-time work may follow when children are older, and then a full-time job may be undertaken again. For women without children, careers may be broken by the need to care for relatives, usually parents. Many women also interweave involvement in community affairs and voluntary work around, for example, the school, the tenants' association, a political campaign or a religious organization. As partners, mothers, workers, providers, carers and activists, we witness women juggling many different roles, demands and tasks. As women, they have to be adaptable and resourceful within a volatile and complex mix of domestic activity and paid and unpaid employment (Patricia Allat *et al.*, 1987). Whatever this mix, the family, friendships, caring relationships and 'the home' represent major areas of investment. This, as Dorothy Jerrome, Sheila Peace and Gillian Dalley all assert, changes little in the postwork phase of later life, providing a strong thread of continuity and stability. Friendship is an important resource in later life. Many women have built strong networks of friends that are not, unlike many men's friendships, dependent on the workplace and thus at risk to dissolution on retirement.

From a broad feminist perspective, the contributors to this book have offered evidence that the sexual division of labour critically influences women's lives right across the life course. The major responsibility which women typically have for unpaid work in the home, and the lack of value placed on this work, creates and maintains unequal access to resources of all kinds. Dulcie Groves (Chapter 3) has shown us how women in old age tend to bear the brunt of a labour market structure which materially rewards those who remain in long-term continuous employment, i.e. primarily men. Moyra Sidell (Chapter 4) draws attention to the different views GPs hold of their male and female patients and the negative gender-role stereotyping which effects their treatment, particularly in relation to mental health. Miriam Bernard and Kathy Meade (Chapter 8) describe the ongoing difficulty women often have in carving out leisure time of their own. The unequal treatment of women has a marked effect on the choices available to them in later life, their ability to participate fully in society, and to maintain autonomy and independence. The chapters on giving and receiving care, and on living environments, amplify this message.

Nevertheless, a significant percentage of older women will face transitions and new situations which may mark off old age from earlier periods in the life course. Change in health status is one example. Moyra Sidell's interviews with older women indicate that while assessing their general health as good or reasonably good, many elderly women report a considerable amount of illness. Statistical evidence certainly shows that older women suffer from more chronic illness than any other age group (see p.70). For individual women, declining health and mobility may have a very pronounced effect on the quality of their lives. Coping with bereavement, and perhaps most particularly the death of a partner, may also have a significant impact. On the other hand, many women report positive experiences in this postmenopause, postwork phase in their lives. New freedoms, new opportunities and new roles may become available.

Dependence, independence and interdependence

A number of stereotypes of women in old age have been challenged throughout the book, including the negative image of women as dependent. This view is linked to a stereotype of older people that portrays them as frail and helpless economic burdens on society. While many older women are reliant on state benefits, it is not old age which is responsible but socially constructed inequalities in income (see p.57). The very word retirement conjures up notions of becoming 'non-productive' and hence dependent (see p.148). So too can presentations of statistical information. Moyra Sidell cites an OPCS study that indicates that 63 per cent of women between 65 and 74 years of age experience long-term health problems that might limit activity. Turned on its head this information gives more cause for optimism, i.e. that 37 per cent of this group of older women are not limited in any way (see p.70). This partial perspective on old age ignores the fact that the majority of older women are in relatively good health, managing their own lives and actively contributing to society.

As many researchers have pointed out, no individual is totally independent. Human beings are all interdependent on each other for support throughout their lives. Given that 'dependence' suggests an unequal distribution of power, and 'independence' is associated with freedom of choice and autonomy, it comes as no surprise that it is a prime concern of older people to assert and maintain their independence.

Disability may dictate greater reliance on help with certain tasks, regardless of age. However, older people give as well as receive, as Clare Wenger (1984) stresses: 'there are more elderly people providing help of one sort or another than there are receiving help'. In Chapter 5 Dorothy Jerrome emphasizes the transactions that go on between the generations in the family. The assumed dependency of older on younger is not a foregone conclusion, as is clearly illustrated by the grandparenting role. Another area which may need rethinking is the links that women have with their offspring. There is already some evidence that adult children are remaining in the home of their parents for longer or returning after marriage break-ups. While some women may welcome this, others may long for the freedom of the 'empty nest'.

Diversity and difference

While we have indicated that there are essential differences in the way women as a group and men as a group experience old age, we have also pointed out that it is unwise to generalize about 'older women'. Older women certainly have much in common because of their gender, but they are not a homogeneous group. There are many differences between them that may either exacerbate or ameliorate their situation. These include age cohorts, class, ethnicity, sexual orientation, marital status and household composition.

Membership of a particular age cohort, for example, may have a significant influence on later life. Those women who were brought up in the Depression are illustrative. They are likely to have had less good health care and nutrition than subsequent generations who had the benefit of a National Health Service. Jewish women too, who as young women fled to the UK from Nazi Germany, experienced the deaths of many of their relatives and friends. This has had a profound effect not only on that generation's mental health but on their friendship and kin networks (Jewish Women in London Group, 1989). Another example is women who worked in what used to be thought of as male jobs in the First and Second World Wars, performed them well and enjoyed newly acquired financial independence and status gained from their economic contribution to running their households. There was widespread resentment when these jobs were reclaimed by men after the Second World War, as happened for example in housing management (Marion Brion and Anthea Tinker, 1980). Such employment experiences may have contributed to this cohort's perception of themselves as subordinate to men.

Despite the difficulties of assigning class to elderly women (see p.12), class differences appear to explain some variations between women, for example in their health status and their access to income in old age. The association between higher socio-economic status and good health has proved to be strong for both older women and men (see p.76). A similar relation is evident with respect to income in later life. Single women from professional and managerial backgrounds are also markedly better off than their single or married sisters who worked in manual jobs.

All too little is known about the current situation, wishes and expectations of elderly people from black and minority ethnic groups, let alone those of women. From the small-scale studies referred to throughout the book, it is clear that there *are* differences and similarities both between older people from black and minority ethnic groups and between them and older white people in terms of personal resources and access to services. Experience of racism and white ethnocentric service provision exacerbates the situation for minority ethnic older people (see pp.76,79 and 121). However, diversity among older black women, as among older women in general, must be acknowledged and attempts to treat them as a homogeneous group should be resisted.

The different life experiences of older lesbian women also need to be acknowledged (see pp.99–103). For example, the impact of having to deny their sexuality, the lack of recognition of their relationships and the lack of rights for lesbian compared with heterosexual married couples is only beginning to be articulated.

Marital status is also shown to be a significant differentiating factor. For instance, widowed and never-married older people, who are in the main women, have a far greater probability of living in a residential home than those who are married. Older married women may also be financially better off if they have access to their husband's income. By contrast, poorer widows may be in a more vulnerable position, surviving on a low income and feeling a lack of security living on their own. On the other hand, women who have never married may have built up their own independent income and, through living alone, may have developed friendship networks and coping strategies (see p.93).

Finally, the support and constraints of the particular household to which older women belong must be taken into account. Older married women who are physically or mentally impaired are mostly cared for by their husbands. However in different circumstances spouses may constrain the activities of their wives. Upon their husband's retirement, some women report considerable disruption as he tries to take greater control over how she spends her time (see pp.158–9). Housing tenure is also relevant. On the one hand, home ownership can be burdensome yet, as a significant form of wealth-holding, it can enhance older women's autonomy and control over their finances, especially in relation to residential care options (see pp.133–4).

An agenda for change: quality and equality

A recurring message throughout the book has been that change for future cohorts of older women depends on changes in the status of women in general. Without the creation of greater social and economic equality between men and women, it is difficult to see how individual women will be able to maximize their life choices as they

age. The disadvantaged position that many older women find themselves in today needs to be confronted. Poverty, poor housing and
lack of access to appropriate services must not be underrated.

Our agenda for change is not intended to be a comprehensive
'shopping list'. Rather, we outline some fundamental demands,
backed by concrete suggestions. These demands centre around:

- valuing caring responsibilities
- ensuring equal opportunities in employment
- preventing income poverty in later life
- responding to the needs of older women

Caring responsibilities

'. . . and I retired. And I went to India, when I came back my husband
was seriously ill. So eight years I worked for my husband, I didn't do
anything else . . . it was very hard work . . .'

(Charanjit)

Caring is still primarily a woman's responsibility and is still largely
unrewarded both in terms of financial recompense and status.
Motherhood and caring commitments, like inequalities in the workplace, have a depressing effect on women's earning power. This has
repercussions in old age (see pp.48–9). If the 'feminization of poverty' is to be halted, let alone rolled back, the valuing of productive
(paid) relative to reproductive (unpaid) work needs to be renegotiated.

There is an unresolved contradiction between the expectation that
women will continue to carry out unpaid caring work within the
family and official encouragement and economic pressure for them
to participate in the labour market. Current government policies
around care in the community and pensions policies amply illustrate
this tension. The former assumes a reserve of informal carers, probably women, yet the latter is premised on responsibility for generating
income for old age through paid work, and contributions to retirement pension schemes. While it has to be said that there has been
some acknowledgement of the economic value to society of caring
through, for example, state retirement pension credits for those
claiming child benefit or caring for certain categories of disabled
people, there has not been any fundamental shift away from
rewarding only those who participate in the labour market. Nor have
we seen much movement towards equal sharing between women and
men in household labour or caring. This failure does, and will continue to have, an enormous impact on the material resources available to all women, and particularly older women.

Equal opportunities in employment

'. . . *Well for the likes of us they weren't really preparing you for anything other than to go and work in the mills. Because you never thought . . . everybody we knew, they worked in the mills. And it was only the better-off people who could hope for an office job . . . And I suppose at that time we just took it for granted that that was our lot . . .*'

(Ray)

Women's employment patterns, as has been indicated, are still profoundly affected by their caring roles in the home. Characteristically women have interrupted records of paid employment and are over-represented in low-waged, part-time work in a narrow range of gender-segregated occupations. Moreover, women are underrepresented at senior levels within most organizations including the civil service, health service and local government. A recent survey of Directors of Social Services, for example, showed that only 12 per cent were women (Nottage, 1991). In some professions the proportion is even smaller (Gibb, 1990). Unfortunately, strategies to tackle sex discrimination in the labour market [the Sex Discrimination Act, 1975; the Equal Pay Act (Amended), 1984] have, to date, had only a limited impact.

For older women workers age discrimination is an added barrier, particularly if they are rejoining the labour market after a long absence (Lazcko and Phillipson, 1991; Catherine Itzin and Chris Phillipson, in press). Many of the traditional 'women's occupations' such as secretarial, reception and shop work seek to recruit young 'attractive' women so that it is not uncommon to see job advertisements stating an age preference for people of 35 and under (EOC, 1989). Equally problematic are employers' demands for previous or recent experience, and a general failure to recognize skills developed through domestic or voluntary unpaid work. Programmes which give 'women returners' confidence and new skills for rejoining the labour market should be more widely available. Education and training opportunities that might enable women to develop new careers from midlife onwards, are still few and far between.

Social policies around 'retirement' and pension ages also have a significant influence on women's employment careers (Fennell *et al.*, 1988). As a result of pressure from the European Community, consultation is underway in the UK on options for the equalization of state pension ages at either 60, 63 or 65, or for a flexible decade of retirement from age 60 to 70, with a 'normal' pensionable age for both sexes to be set somewhere between 60 and 65 (DSS, 1991a). The first proposal clearly protects women's existing position. The last option would only increase the choices for women if they were able to choose to work until 70, or draw a pension at any time between 60 and 70 that is adequate to live on. With the available evidence of ageism in employment, any such flexible retirement policy would need to be backed by age discrimination legislation in order to extend to older workers legal protection from, for example, unfair dismissal on the grounds of age. Given the interconnection between access to financial resources in early and later life, improvement in women's position in the paid workplace has to be a priority.

Income poverty in later life

'. . . *I've always had part-time jobs. So I never paid for a bigger pension. Sorry now, but I manage. I get by. I say to myself there's nothing I want in a hurry. I could do with a new three-piece, I could do with a new carpet, I could do with a new mattress, things like that. But I don't really need them. You see what I mean . . .*'

(Olga)

Currently, income levels in later life are determined largely by each individual's ability to defer income gained from paid employment. In the absence of a guaranteed basic income for all, those who forgo earnings so as to carry out unpaid work lose out (Wicks, 1987). Redress for older women in the future depends on how closely income in retirement continues to be linked to previous paid employment and to pensions policies.

Over the last ten years government policies have emphasized the desirability for individuals to make financial provision for their own old age in addition to the basic state retirement pension, notably by means of second-tier portable personal pensions. Such policies are intended to counter reliance on the SERPS. But, personal pensions have several disadvantages, not least the fact that the eventual amount of pension cannot be predicted. Women's payments to personal pension schemes are adversely affected by absence(s) from the labour market and part-time earnings. A better alternative might well be membership of an occupational pension scheme that offers a guaranteed level of benefit linked to final salary, and fully index-linked against inflation. However, lower paid women may find themselves offered inferior employers' schemes where the final pension is linked to invested contributions only, and is not fully index-linked. Such occupational pensions are, like personal pensions, based on the expectation of continuous employment. If this approach to income provision in later life is to prevail for the foreseeable future, the government could, at the very least, consider ways of encouraging more employers to offer good occupational pension schemes to lower paid and part-time workers.

Policies that enable women to build up entitlement to a full basic state retirement pension by means of contributions and credits offer a better option for women. But only on the proviso that the level of that pension is itself adequate. There is evidence that state provision could be significantly improved if the financial incentives currently given by the state to the private pension schemes were transferred back to the state (Reddin and Pilch, 1985). The original SERPS scheme was the best second-tier provision yet devised for women who did not have access to a good occupational pension scheme. It recognized periods of absence from the labour force and fluctuating earnings by basing the eventual pension on a contributor's 'best twenty years'. There is no reason why a future government should not devise a replacement that could match the best occupational or personal schemes.

Another option is a really adequate basic pension available as a citizen's right and funded from taxation (Midwinter, 1985). As Dulcie Groves (1991) has suggested, we need to question 'to what extent an individualistic and workplace based approach to financial provision for old age, let alone any arrangements which depend on the continuation of married status, are really in women's best interests, given the economic uncertainty of many women's lives' (p.59). A citizen's pension could recompense older women now for all the low-paid and unpaid work that they have carried out and indeed continue to carry out.

There is considerable debate about what might constitute an adequate minimum level of income for older people. The labour movement, backed by national pensioners' organizations, has tried to quantify this, and has campaigned for years for an immediate commitment to a single person's state retirement pension level of not less than one-third of the average gross earnings for a single person. In 1992 this would give a pension of over £93 as opposed to the current level of £54.15. But even this target amount still assumes some additional allowance towards housing costs. Peter Townsend (1979) talks of a 'participation standard' below which it is not possible to take part in the ordinary life of society. To date however, little research has been carried out on what this income level might be for older people. However what is clear is that the current government is not likely to countenance such an increase in the basic state pension. Nor does it seem likely to restore the relationship between the state pension increase and whatever is the more favourable rise in average earnings or prices. Since 1980, the linking of pension increases to prices alone has resulted in a steady devaluing of the basic pension. Many older women, dependent entirely on state provision, have not shared in the rising living standards that have resulted from the increase in the real value of wages. This, at the very least, should be rectified.

With little hope of any foreseeable rise in the level of the state pension older women, who have no other means of generating income, will have no choice but to rely heavily on other forms of publicly funded financial support, e.g. social security and housing benefits. These benefits top up the basic pension but are means-tested and linked to a subsistence definition of income maintenance. Means-testing itself is problematic, and is intensely disliked by most older people for its connections with 'National Assistance', charity and the stigma of failing to provide for oneself. Moreover, the very existence of this poverty safety-net sidesteps the fundamental demand, which we endorse, of ensuring that older women (and older men) have access to an adequate income as of right.

Concessionary and subsidized services also make a significant contribution to the income support of older women. Many of these were introduced by local authorities in response to the needs and poverty of older people in their communities. They are maintained at the discretion of each Council and, consequently, vary significantly from authority to authority. These concessions include, for example, free bus passes or reduced fare schemes, free or subsidized home helps, concessions for adult education classes, or use of leisure facilities. But local government itself is under enormous pressure to cut spending to the extent that all these collective provisions, if not already reduced, are in serious danger of erosion. The choices are stark. Right across the country there is evidence of charges being introduced or increased, of greater means-testing and/or cuts in the total amount of service provision. Yet all this is taking place in the context of decreases in the real value of the pension. For too many older women, there is little cause for optimism.

The needs of older women

'. . . *Well what I want for myself in old age is to stay in my own home as long as possible. Well, till I snuff it. I would not want to go in a home—I like my independence, and I like to watch what I want on television, and I want to turn it off and read . . . And if help is needed then I expect to be helped by Social Services—a warden or somebody coming in—a home help, or whatever. But I don't want to be taken out of my own home . . .*'

(Ray)

Security, autonomy, independence, a sense of purpose and friendship networks, have all emerged from the preceding chapters as key ingredients for a good quality life for older women. However without adequate financial resources at their disposal many older women's choices are severely constrained. As a result the range of support services and opportunities that might enable older women to maintain, let alone enhance, their quality of life, have been determined largely by service providers, be they in the public, private, or voluntary sector.

We identify four interdependent issues that must be addressed if older women are to achieve their expressed goals. These are:

- equality of access
- the development of user-centred services
- a holistic approach
- preventative measures

To illustrate each of these issues we have chosen examples relating to the health needs of older women. But, it is important to stress that equivalent instances could be readily drawn from an exploration of other needs in older women's lives, whether for accommodation or practical support, for recognition, for social contact or for leisure. While our focus is on older women, we recognize that many of the changes we recommend will benefit older men too.

First, we urge service providers to examine their policies and practices in order to ensure equality of access. Overt age discrimination against older women is clearly evident, for instance in current health policies on breast and cervical cancer screening. The incidence of breast cancer rises steadily as women get older, yet only women aged between 50 and 64 are invited for screening. Some 40 per cent of deaths from cervical cancer in England occur in women over 65, yet again screening is restricted to younger women. There is considerable debate about the value or otherwise of 'whole population screening' but, 'that little is known about the natural history of the cancer of the cervix does not seem to have been an obstacle to the introduction of screening programmes for younger women' (Astrid Fletcher, 1992).

In both these examples, older women are the visible victims of unequal treatment. However they also experience indirect discrimination. Too often we hear older women reporting the response 'What do you expect at your age?' when they raise their health concerns (see p.78). A cycle of disadvantage is perpetuated: such ageist professional attitudes ration older people's access to services and, in turn, reinforce older people's low expectations of their own health and wellbeing, and their confidence to explore the options that might be available to them. This can be especially true for certain older women with no available friends or relatives to advocate on their behalf.

The provision of information is one key to redressing the impact of such ageism. There is, without doubt, an increasing amount of information about what can contribute to good physical and mental health in later life, about what people can do to improve their own health and what services and facilities may be available. Yet as one recent study reported: 'Very often elderly people have either not heard about it, understood it, accepted it or acted upon it' (King's Fund, 1988, p.29). Or, as another researcher succinctly puts it, many older people suffer from 'a famine among plenty' (Christine Mullins, 1990).

While the availability of up-to-date, practical and non-patronizing information is essential, it is not, on its own, a sufficient response to the problem of access. How service providers perceive older women and their needs, along with how older women themselves are consulted and involved in decisions about these needs, are also central concerns. We return to these issues later in the chapter.

The second issue which has to be addressed focuses on the development of services which are user-centred, and more specifically, women-centred. Throughout the 1980s and 1990s consumerism has become fashionable. The NHS and Community Care Act (1990) makes many references to consumers, customers and clients and stresses the importance of involving people in devising their own 'package of care'. The Patients Charter, in the company of the Citizen's Charter and a myriad of similar statements emanating from public and private sector organizations, endorses concepts of customer choice and the right to quality services. The message is clear, but the process and desired outcome of shifting the balance of power towards those using the services, and away from those providing them, is proving problematic. At least this seems to be so, if the experience of older women to date is any guide. The availability of financial resources, and their allocation both within and between the major service providers, is forwarded as the principal, but not the only, stumbling block.

For example, the evidence which Moyra Sidell outlines in Chapter 4 indicates that older women suffer from more chronic conditions than men or any other age group. Rheumatoid arthritis is one such condition. It can cause considerable pain and serious mobility problems that can make going out unaided, or managing household tasks in the home, very difficult. Joint replacements, and especially hip replacements, have proved to be most successful medical interventions. Yet the waiting time for such operations on the NHS has been anything from six months to four years or longer. Acute healthcare still dominates health-service provision, despite efforts to shift the balance towards the aptly described 'Cinderella services' for those older women with non-life-threatening conditions.

Alongside the preventable suffering and loss of independence for every older woman forced to wait for a hip replacement, are issues regarding the transfer of costs onto other services. During this waiting time the local authority may have to provide equipment (from walking aids to hand rails and raised toilet seats) to enable the older woman to manage at home, a home help and meals on wheels. Her

family, friends and neighbours may also be called for additional practical support such as transport to help her maintain her social contacts. The cost-effectiveness of this scenario, for both the individual
and the public purse, merits closer scrutiny.

However, in other situations, it is the assumptions that underpin
the way a service is provided that may render it insensitive to the
needs of older women. Stereotypical perceptions that all older
women are white, or that their families should be ready and able to
offer support, or that they are unable or unwilling to make decisions
about their own care, have a strong influence on the quality of the
service. Shah Ebrahim (1992) graphically illustrates this through the
experience of one older woman and her family:

> 'A Bangladeshi woman had a stroke which left her badly paralysed and
> unable to speak. A social worker saw the family, and her children were
> used as interpreters as no hospital interpreter was available. The family
> was asked if they would take her home and they replied with the literal
> reply "Yes, they would be able to take their mother home." What they
> meant was they would be able to physically transport her from hospital
> to home . . . Much to the delight of the hospital staff she went home and
> from their point of view it was a "successful" discharge, but for the family
> it was a nightmare. No one had explained . . . The community nursing
> service had assumed the family could cope because there were enough of
> them, and the social services had a policy of not providing support if there
> were other people living in the house . . .' (pp.170–71).

This leads us to our third demand, which is for a holistic approach
to responding to older women's needs. Maintaining good health for
example, is not simply about medical interventions. The ability to
stay active and independent may well depend as much on the local
bus service or Dial-a-Ride and adult education classes as it does on
prescribed medication for an underlying health condition. For each
older woman there are inextricable links between her personal and
material circumstances (e.g. health status, race, income, housing or
friendship network), and the support she might want from the
healthcare system and other services (e.g. home helps, public transport, sheltered housing schemes, or social or leisure opportunities).
As we saw earlier, a decision by one service provider (not to perform
enough hip-replacement operations, or to move patients back as
quickly as possible into the community) has a knock-on effect on
other providers (local authorities and social networks).

At both a strategic planning and at an individual level improved
coordination and collaboration would seem to be a prerequisite if
older women are to find appropriate, flexible, yet comprehensive
solutions to their needs. Under community-care policies, joint planning between social services and health services is a primary objective. But we question whether this goes far enough. Key contributors

to enabling older women to remain independent, for example hous-ing, leisure and education departments, transport and town planners, may not be part of the process. Environmental solutions, such as designing and equipping accommodation with low-cost aids such as ramps or bath rails, ensuring that local shops and post offices stay open, making the most of local community centres for keep-fit sessions, a lunch club and a mobile chiropody service, or putting more accessible buses onto the roads, are as much part of the fabric of living in the community as home-care services. Mechanisms for facilitating this sort of 'neighbourhood-based' planning, in partner-ship with older women, need to be developed.

Finally, we would argue for a shift of focus and resources into preventive activity. The treatment of osteoporosis, another health condition that differentially affects older women as opposed to older men, offers some clear messages. It is estimated that, at any one time, approximately 20 per cent of all orthopaedic beds are occupied by women with hip fractures due to osteoporosis. In 1988 the hospital cost alone of osteoporotic hip fractures was in the region of £500 million (Office of Health Economics, 1990; Smith, 1992). Yet there has been little priority given to research into both screening and the relative benefits of possible preventive therapies such as HRT, cal-cium in the diet or weight-bearing exercise (Melanie Henwood, 1990a; Smith, 1992). As with arthritis, the failure to respond appro-priately has both individual and social costs.

On the other hand there are data available on the value of physical activity programmes to build up muscle strength for older men (Adrianne Hardman, 1991). This suggests that a 10 to 20 per cent improvement in strength effectively postpones strength-related thre-sholds of disability (e.g. to use public transport) for at least ten to twenty years. If older women were to participate in similar activities, there appears to be no reason why it would not have an equivalent impact on their quality of life. However, most GPs are not trained to give the specialist exercise advice needed, nor do they have the resources to support and monitor progress. Yet, the exercise experts who are most likely to be found in leisure centres or in adult edu-cation do not, in general, offer extensive provision for older people, nor have formal links with the health promotion arm of the health service.

From a brief exploration of these four priorities for improving responses to the health needs of older women, it is evident that some quite fundamental questions have to be asked about the design, quality, availability and accessibility of all service provision. The state is the major provider of health, material and supportive resources, and we have seen that within this provision older women are dis-advantaged. But, if state provision for older women were reduced the inequalities would increase. Since many older women lack their own resources, any attack on collective provision will have a strongly negative impact on their wellbeing. Rather, we argue for a strengthened role for the state at both a national and local level in ensuring that the needs of older women are systematically met (Sara Arber and Jay Ginn, 1991b; Joanna Bornat *et al.*, 1985).

Action for change

In the context of a 'prejudiced world', combatting ageist and sexist attitudes and practices is likely to be difficult. Valuing the experience of older women suggests that we should rethink many of the social structures and policies that affect day-to-day life in old age. Ultimately, such change is about a shift in power, status and resources that, if the history of the struggles around race and gender repeats itself, will not be willingly conceded.

We turn now to considering how older women themselves, older people's organizations, as well as professional and academic bodies, are contributing, and might contribute to this process. Throughout this section we draw on illustrative examples collated from a questionnaire we sent to over one hundred groups and organizations (Jean Shapiro, 1989, pp.573–83). Contact addresses can be found in Appendix 1 (see p.191).

Older women speaking up for themselves

There are small signs in Britain of groups of older women who are actively engaged in campaigning for improvements in older women's lives. For example, the Pensioners' Link Older Women's Project in London, under the banner of 'Older Women—old, proud and powerful', brings together older women from different backgrounds and cultures to discuss and campaign around issues of concern. A working group of older women plans and monitors the project's initiatives. Since 1985 it has, amongst other things, helped to set up borough-based older women's groups, and held conferences for older women on themes such as transport, housing, Europe, and the concerns of black and minority ethnic older women. Six hundred members receive their quarterly newsletter. The Older Feminist Network, which has a national focus, also produces a newsletter. This self-financed network holds monthly workshops in London to enable its members to be better informed, and equipped to raise the concerns of older women in whatever other organizations they may be involved with. The Older Lesbian Network operates in a similar way.

Through the efforts of these groups, older women's voices are beginning to be heard within women's organizations and the pensioners' movement. In April 1992, the National Pensioners Convention (an umbrella organization of pensioners groups) for the first time acknowledged discrimination against older women. Amendments were made to the Pensioners' Charter to include demands for the equalization of the state pension age and for flexible retirement with a basic state pension from the age of 60. These were subsequently endorsed at the European Senior Citizens' Parliament in Luxembourg. In May 1992, the Older Feminist Network, backed by the Older Women's Project, succeeded in gaining the commitment of the National Alliance Of Women's Organizations (NAWO) to campaign for breast screening for older women over 65 on the same basis as for younger women. NAWO also endorsed support for the pension rights of part-time workers and carers.

Nevertheless, it is worth stressing again that much of the energy and enthusiasm of the women's movement has been focused on younger women (see pp.14–16). As Olive Stevenson (1987) has pointed out, 'Feminists themselves have been criticized for the length of time it has taken them to espouse the cause of their elder sisters' (p.6). This accusation can also be directed at the pensioners movement for its failure to take on gender issues. Neither the National Pensioners' Convention, nor the more militant Pensioners' Rights Campaign, nor the more middle-class Association of Retired Persons (ARP) have comprehensive policies that reflect women's disadvantaged position in terms of money or health, let alone inequalities within the home. Their charters demand improvements that will affect all old people but that ignore differences arising from race or gender. If introduced, such improvements will certainly make older women's lives better, but they will fail to redress any of the inequalities that we have described in this book. One way forward for both national women's and pensioners' organizations may be through the adoption of the EURAG (European Federation for the Welfare of the Elderly) Statement on the Rights and Needs of Older Women (see p.194, Appendix 2).

This situation in the UK contrasts markedly with that in the USA. There the Older Women's League (OWL) campaigns on older women's issues as part of the National Organization of Women. Maggie Kuhn and the Gray Panthers have also promoted older women's interests, stressing the interdependence between young and old people and the integration of older people into the mainstream of community life. Furthermore, the American Association of Retired Persons (AARP) has a specific Women's Initiative. A network of trained volunteer spokeswomen seek out opportunities to educate and influence AARP members, community leaders and policy makers. While this may be no excuse for their neglect of older women's issues, it has to be said that the British organizations do not have access to the same level of resources and, in comparison with their American counterparts, operate on shoestring budgets. AARP, with 50 million members, has a strong financial base and hence a sound foundation for building a campaigning organization.

Empowering older women

A key aim of the three older women's groups described above is to empower older women with the necessary knowledge, skills, and confidence to make informed choices and to contribute to decision-making that affects their lives at an individual, local and national level. An allied goal is to share information and experience about the services and facilities that are available, and to offer opportunities for older women who may lack the confidence to develop new skills and try out new activities.

In some areas, informal networks of interested professionals have made links with older women locally to encourage this process. This has been particularly evident in the field of health promotion (see pp.277–8). For example, in Tyneside and Gateshead a group of women workers in the health service, community health projects and voluntary organizations (Women Working with Older Women), has come together to develop health promotion initiatives with women aged 40 and over. Since 1989 they have organized: a Forty Plus Festival (with workshops on keeping fit, dance, breast screening, HRT, yoga and relaxation, massage, etc.); 'taster' days at two leisure centres; and a half-day event, 'Women's Minds Matter', designed around mental health and emotional wellbeing. In Manchester a similar network, brought together under Age Concern England's Age-Well Campaign, held a conference on Older Women and Health. The exchange of ideas here has led to a closer collaboration between older women and health workers in setting up new services and health promotion activities. The Sports Council's '50+ and all to play for' campaign has also encouraged the development of new opportunities in physical recreation for older women. The Forty Something club in Welwyn Garden City and the Women's 'We Can Do It' group in Harlow are two examples.

On a broader educational front there are other pioneering examples. In London the Older Women's Education Group has, since 1988, held seven study days on subjects ranging from media images of older women, the challenge of racism, work and leisure, campaigning, and the quality of life. Between 40 and 100 older women attend each event. Here, older women work in partnership with Birkbeck College, University of London and the Education Resources Unit for Older People at the City Lit. Another collaboration, between the self-organized Life Long Learning/University of the Third Age Groups and the University of Central Lancashire, has resulted in the establishment of a bursary to enable a woman over the age of 60, without previous higher education, to study for an undergraduate degree. At an international level, a joint local authority/European Commission initiative, the European Older Women's Project, is making links between older women in Lewisham and eight European countries. Through visits to each other's countries, groups of older women are deepening their understanding of women's position across different cultures and societies, and learning about alternative ways of meeting their needs.

Unfortunately, there are fewer signs of initiatives designed to empower older women within the mainstream of adult education provision. What is on offer is still largely a 'women's curriculum' of craft and home-based skills such as patchwork, canework or cake decoration. Some feminist educationalists argue that this focus on domestically useful knowledge 'enables women to become more satisfied consumers of their own oppression', and confirms their role within the home to the detriment of their personal development and to the exclusion of other roles (Nell Keddie in Jane Thompson, 1983, p.84). If education is regarded as part of the process of social change there is much that could be learned from the approach of the learning programmes designed to enable younger working-class women, and black women in particular, to broaden their horizons, gain confidence and new skills. Patricia Allat (1990), for example, argues the case for assertiveness training for older women in the light of the skills they need to deal with professionals, be it around entitlement to benefits, or gaining access to services. She poses a goal for older women, individually and collectively, 'to be able to come away from an encounter without feeling that somehow you have "lost"; that you have been able to set out your position and are not merely a cipher, a burden, or someone who can be easily tucked away or become invisible to others' (p.4).

A corollary to the empowerment of older women is the possibility of influencing the decision-making bodies that affect their lives. The health and personal social services, for example, are littered with attempts to involve users in the planning, or delivery or monitoring of services. In a recent nationwide survey, Peter Beresford and Suzy Croft (1990) found that just under one-third of Social Services Departments, and nearly half of the voluntary organizations, had formal policies about the involvement of users. However this study cautioned that in many instances, contact with users and potential users only masqueraded as consultation. In reality, the service provider approached the community to give information about, or seek support for, a course of action, but had little intention of modifying it. Genuine consultation actively seeks the advice of users, and at best tries to involve them both in identifying the problem and working out the solution. Such participation requires service providers to think about service users in a new way and to value their perspective. To date, there is very limited documentation of older people's role in such developments and even less about the particular input of older women (Jocelyn Cornwell, 1989; Liz Winn, 1990; Tony Carter and Caroline Nash, in press).

Educating professionals

The discussion above leads us to consider just how appropriate is the training received by many of the professional groups who work with older women. It is clear from the previous chapters that the attitudes shown towards older women leave a great deal to be desired. It may well be that this generation of older women is accustomed to being deferential towards, for example, the medical profession.

Unfortunately, very little is taught about either the ageing process, or the experience of being old, in the initial training of many professionals such as doctors, social workers and nurses. This inevitably means that their perceptions and attitudes are coloured by those older people whom they meet in the course of their working day. These are more likely to be older people who are sick or who are facing problems with money, housing or caring responsibilities. They are less likely to meet older people who are managing well and leading relatively active and satisfying lives. This may help to account for the prevailing pathological view of old age which sees only disease, disability, dependency and poverty.

If little is taught about the positive aspects of ageing even less explores gender issues in later life. For example, Catherine Rees (1991) found in her recent study of social workers, old women and female carers, that much social work theory and practice does not have a gender perspective nor a sensitivity towards specific problems which older women encounter. This confirms the earlier findings by Janet Finch and Dulcie Groves (1985).

Olive Stevenson (1987), among others, argues for greater investment in education and training for all staff who care for elderly people, starting with an examination of attitudes. Such training needs to acknowledge the tension between increasing professional expertise and knowledge, while retaining a commitment to increase the power of older people to control their own lives (Phillipson, 1990). Phillipson advocates a curriculum that includes examining the role of social processes (ageism, passive forms of care, financial and other forms of disadvantage) in producing and maintaining dependency in later life, and developing skills around empowerment and maximizing self-determination. This would counterbalance the current problem-centred training with its emphasis on decline and loss of ability. Additionally, he asserts the desirability of involving older people themselves in the delivery of such programmes.

On the positive side, we have witnessed in the last five years a major expansion in the numbers of certificate, postgraduate and post-qualifying courses in gerontology that have been built on this approach. These programmes attract students from a wide range of professional backgrounds such as social workers, residential care staff and health-service personnel. Multidisciplinary courses are particularly likely to enhance understanding of issues of gender. Some, like Keele University, include specific modules on women and later life. The task now is to ensure that a more holistic study both of ageing and of gender is incorporated into all the basic professional training of those who work with older people.

Developing legislation and codes of practice

Alongside the strategies outlined above we also acknowledge the value of a collective, legally enforceable framework for tackling age and sex discrimination. Earlier in the chapter we commented on the limited success to date of the Sex Discrimination Act (1975) and the Equal Pay Act [(Amended), 1984] in achieving equal opportunities for women in employment. Nevertheless, such legislation does provide a statutory safeguard against sex discrimination and gives individuals the right to seek legal remedies through the courts.

We support the demand for an Age Discrimination Act, which would follow the lines of the Sex Discrimination legislation and the Race Relations Act 1976 (Evelyn McEwen, 1990). This could, in the words of those Acts, make age discrimination 'unlawful in employment, training and related matters, in education, in the provision of goods and services and in the disposal and management of premises'. Under such legislation the right to work would depend on individual ability to do the job; arbitrary age limits for renewing drivers' licences, retiring, donating blood, doing jury service or chairing an Industrial Tribunal amongst other things, would be outlawed. It might also be used to create benchmarks in the range and quality of services that might enable older women to participate equally in the life of the community. The level of provision of transport, of home adaptations, or of leisure opportunities, might be tested under such legislation.

The adoption of Codes of Practice, both by professional organizations and service providers is another useful strategy. For instance, the Code of Practice for the press and media, proposed by the CPA, would commit them to avoid quoting chronological age unless it was properly relevant (Midwinter, 1991b). The Home Life (residential care), Community Life and Leisure Life Codes for local authorities are other examples (CPA, 1984; 1990; 1992). Such codes, however, should specifically promote good practice in relation to gender as well as age.

Extending our understanding of older women's lives

In writing this book we have attempted to provide an overview of what is known about the lives of older women. It is evident that quite a lot is known. Yet on many occasions our contributors have commented that there is inadequate data and, in so doing, have highlighted the directions for further research that builds on our current understanding.

First, there needs to be more work in all the areas we have discussed: research that focuses not only on gender differences, but on variations among women. Much of the information that does exist about older people is not broken down on a gender basis and, conversely, what we know about women is not differentiated by age. More particularly, we know very little about older black and minority ethnic women. Other important differences that merit closer examination include sexual orientation and marital status. Not only do we need to learn more, for example, about the lives of older single women, we need to compare their lives with those, say, of married women, in order to increase our understanding of the diverse ways in which women experience old age.

Second, much of the research cited throughout the book is descriptive. As discussed in Chapter 1, the development of many of the theoretical models for understanding ageing or gender have not been tested in relation to older women (see pp.5–16). These theories need to be scrutinized afresh. As Baba Copper (1988) has argued, 'it should not be impossible to be both a feminist and a gerontologist' although, as she goes on to say:

> 'the two do not seem to coincide with any regularity. There has been a great silence about woman-to-woman ageism. The issues specific to female age have never been incorporated into any feminist list of the twenty most needed changes. A mutually beneficial dialogue between the generations of women is still in the future' (p.60).

We would specifically argue for feminist research that builds on a life-course perspective. It is worth restating here that this approach appears to offer a fruitful way forward with its emphasis on 'the changing individual in a changing society' (Leonie Sugarman, 1986, p.46). It recognizes the importance of individual history and the dynamic interaction between the individual and the environment. It could most usefully enhance our understanding of, for example, women's experience of the transition to retirement, their attitudes towards and preferences for different kinds of services or housing or leisure opportunities, and of being cared for, if necessary, in old age.

Finally, we reiterate the need for more sensitive research methods (see pp.16–18). Qualitative approaches that enable the subjective experience of older women to be heard have the potential to advance our understanding, as many of the small-scale studies we have drawn on testify. This is not to discount the value of gender- and age-differentiated statistical research, but to suggest that both have their place.

Conclusion

'. . . *We've got so many young people today that look at us older ones as if we're something from outer space. They don't realize we built this estate up, we got the telephones, we got the clubs going. We got —you know there was nothing for us at all . . .'*

'. . . *Oh, I've made my own life and as much as my mother kept us under, so did my husband keep me under. My children will never be under their husbands' thumbs like I was . . .'*

(Olga)

It would seem that to be old and a woman is to be in a contradictory position. Older women bear the impact of an ageist and sexist society that forces many of them into poverty and dependence, yet conversely many live relatively satisfying lives and are far from passive victims. Women share similar life experiences and have much in common, but there are many differences between them and the strengths they bring to old age. Society, however, alternately regards them as a 'burden' or as a 'resource'. Their own personal goals are rarely acknowledged, nor is their desire for autonomy, security, a sense of purpose and of enjoyment.

For older women, achievement of this wellbeing lies in fundamental changes that tackle the origins of their disadvantage. Women's position in the home and in the workplace has a critical and cumulative effect on the quality of later life. Women's caring responsibilities across the life course need to be valued and equality of opportunity in employment secured. The income poverty experienced by so many older women will only be ameliorated if the current relation between income, paid employment, unpaid domestic labour and pension policies is radically altered. An adequate basic state pension would be a first step.

Older women rely heavily on public-sector services for healthcare, practical support in the home, housing and leisure opportunities. Any shift from public to private responsibility for community care, for example, and any resulting cuts in public expenditure, have severe gender-specific implications. The majority of frail older people are women. Likewise, the family and neighbour network who are expected to take over are mainly women of the next (younger but not so young) generation. This pressure on women as carers and as care-recipients has to be resisted.

There is much that is good in the services and facilities available to older people but questions have to be asked about how sensitive and responsive they are to the needs of older women. Access to appropriate support and opportunities can be difficult and is often denied. Stereotypical and negative views of older women influence service design and quality. Older women are rarely consulted about how to improve current services or to meet new needs. Increasing the available resources is a necessary response but not the only one. Changes in the way services are developed and delivered are equally important. Investment in staff training that counters the current problem-oriented approach to old age is one way forward. Developing consultative and participatory decision-making processes is another. Codes of practice and antidiscriminatory legislation are also advocated.

All of this agenda can be accomplished. It certainly requires political and popular will and vision. It requires acknowledging the rights of older women to a quality of life based on autonomy, security and fulfilment. Older women know what it is like to be old, but contemporary society does not make it easy for their voices to be heard. Only when the needs of older women have been fully recognized and understood, and the necessary steps taken to ensure that they are met, will it be possible for us to claim that women truly have 'come of age'.

Appendix 1
Women's and older people's organizations

Older women's initiatives

European Older Women's Project (Lewisham)
Lewisham Pensioners Officer
Lewisham Equal Opportunities Unit
Lewisham Town Hall
Catford Broadway
London   SE6 4SW
Tel: 081 659 6000 ext 3200

Older Feminists Network
c/o 54 Gordon Road
London   N3 1EP
Tel: 081 346 1900

Older Lesbian Network
c/o London Women's Centre
Wesley House
4 Wild Court
London   WC2

Older Women's Education Group
c/o EdROP—Education Resources for Older People
The City Lit
6 Bolt Court
London   EC4A 3DQ
Tel: 071 405 2949

Older Women's Project
Manor Gardens Centre
6–9 Manor Gardens
London   N7 6LA
Tel: 071 281 3485

The Winifred Keen Bursary for Women Over 60
Life Long Learning
University of Central Lancashire

Preston   PR1 2TQ
Tel: 0722 892 379

The Women 'We Can Do It' Group
Women's Sports Motivator
Arts and Recreation Services
Latton Bush
Sutton Way
Harlow
Tel: 079 446 417

Women Working with Older Women
c/o Tyneside Women's Health Project
Swinburne House
Swinburne Street
Gateshead   NE8 1AX
Tel: 091 477 7898

40+ Women's Group
Campus West Leisure Division
Welwyn Garden City   AL8 6BX
Tel: 0707 339 211

Women's organizations

National Alliance of Women's Organisations (NAWO)
279–281 Whitechapel Road
London   E1 1BY
Tel: 071 247 7052

Older people's organizations

Age Concern England
1268 London Road
London   SW16 4ER
Tel: 081 679 8000

Age Concern Scotland
54a Fountainbridge
Edinburgh   EH3 9PT
Tel: 031 228 5656

Age Concern Wales
4th Floor
1 Cathedral Road
Cardiff   CF1 9SD
Tel: 0222 371 566

Age Well
Age Concern England (as above)

Association of Retired Persons (ARP)
Parnell House
19–21 Wilton Road
London   SW1V 1LW
Tel: 071 895 8881

Beth Johnson Foundation
64 Princes Road
Hartshill
Stoke-on-Trent   ST4 7JL
Tel: 0782 44036

Centre for Policy on Ageing
25–31 Ironmonger Row
London   EC1V 3QP
Tel: 071 253 1787

National Pensioners Convention
Plot 148
Manorfields
Hunstanton   PE36 5PE
Tel: 0885 534 619

Pensioners' Rights Campaign
Harlington Place
Carlisle   CA1 1HL
Tel: 0228 22681

Pre-Retirement Association
Nodus Centre
University of Surrey
Guildford   GU2 5RY
Tel: 0483 39390

50+ and All To Play For Campaign
Sports Council
16 Upper Woburn Place
London   WC1H 0QP
Tel: 071 388 1277

Appendix 2
Older women in Europe: their needs and rights

At the 12th International Congress of EURAG (The European Federation for the Welfare of The Elderly) held in the Netherlands in May 1988, the following statement about the rights of older women was adopted.

Rights of older women

In Europe the vast majority of the elderly population are women and they have a positive contribution to make to society through their knowledge, experience, creativity and skills. They are a valuable resource that often is unacknowledged. And indeed, the reality of their lives in today's ageist and sexist society is that many are single, alone and living below the poverty line, especially in the more vulnerable higher age groups.

The future will see a rapid increase in this age group who, without economic independence, good housing and preventive and curative health care, could present a heavy burden on society.

However, if present needs are met, this situation could largely be prevented. In some European countries older women are today, in an unprecedented way, finding a voice to articulate these needs.

Older women in other countries need encouragement to voice their needs. Asserting their rights to dignity and a better quality of life will not only improve their own situations, but also that of the men of their own generation. Older women must be enabled to participate in all social planning to meet these needs.

The following are some of the most important rights to which we believe older women are entitled.

1. We affirm the right of all women to security and independence in their later years. To implement this right, governments must provide a level of income which will enable them to live with dignity, through such means as:

    a. Promotion of employment opportunities for older women and programmes to facilitate re-entry into the labour force by older women and adoption of affirmative action plans.

b. A flexible retirement age so that older women who wish either to retire early or to work reduced hours, or who need or wish to continue working beyond the present age of retirement, may have a choice.

c. Upon retirement, a pension adequate to provide a good standard of living. We note that for some women who are not yet old this right is already threatened by lack of adequate pension arrangements.

d. Recognition of the unpaid contribution of the women whose work is within the home, of assisting wives and of rural women, to the nation's economy by inclusion in contributory pension schemes.

e. Special attention to the problems of minority, immigrant and disabled older women.

f. More funds made available from the European Social Fund for training for re-entry to the work force.

2. We affirm the right of older women to affordable housing and a safe environment, accessible by public transport. To implement this right, governments must provide or support—

a. Sufficient housing of good quality in the non-profit sector, and control of the standards of provision in the private sector.

b. A range of alternative living arrangements from independent housing units to various styles of communal households and sheltered living units to avoid the social isolation of single elderly women.

c. Representation of older women in the decision making bodies who create the infrastructure of housing planning, transport, etc.

3. We affirm the right of older women who need care to obtain community support systems, keeping in mind that, in many cases, families are not present, or are not in a position to take care of them.

For those older women who are care-givers to aged parents, spouses, friends, neighbours or other family members, governments should supply economic support and relief, respite care and other services. Older women who are carers should have equal rights to participate in social security and in social innovations.

4. We affirm the right of older women to a health care system which respects their differences, which emphasizes prevention of health problems, access to rehabilitation, which avoids over-medication, and which takes into consideration the realities of the woman's life situation. Older women of the ethnic minority groups have particular health needs which the health care system must meet. Older women should be given the opportunity to participate in decisions regarding

their health, and their proposals should be formally recorded. The formation of self-help groups should be encouraged.

To achieve these rights, older women must have a full voice in decision-making at all levels of governmental organisations. Where such bodies do not presently exist, official commission should be established to give attention to the needs of older women. Organizations carrying out activities for and with older women should be given financial support. Special regard should be paid to the education of women themselves, the public and members of the government on the need for changes in attitudes and traditional sex-roles. Whilst research is needed on the situation of all older people, it is necessary for more attention to be paid by researchers to the situation of older women, keeping in mind the differences in age, life-style and socio-economic position and needs.

Finally, we call on all governments to take the necessary steps to implement the existing recommendations concerning the position of elderly women laid down in the documents of the EEC, the European Parliament, the Council of Europe, ILO, and the United Nations, especially the UN Vienna International Plan of Action on Ageing 1982 and the Nairobi Forward Looking Strategies for the Advancement of Women 1985.

References

Abrams, M. (1978). *Beyond Three Score and Ten—A First Report on a Survey of the Elderly*. Age Concern England, London.

Abrams, M. (1980). *Beyond Three-score and Ten: A Second Report on a Survey of the Elderly*. Age Concern England, London.

Action for Health (1988). *Initiation in Local Communities*. Community Projects Foundation, London.

Adelman, M. (Ed.) (1986). *Long Time Passing: Lives of Older Lesbians*. Alyson Publications, Boston, MA.

Ade-Ridder, L. (1990). Sexual and marital equality among older married couples. In *Family Relationships in Later Life*, second edition, Brubaker, T. (Ed.), pp.48–67. Sage Publications Inc., Newbury Park, CA.

Advisory Council for Adult and Continuing Education (1982). *Adults: Their Educational Experience and Needs*. ACACE, Leicester.

Age Concern England (1974). *The Attitudes of the Retired and Elderly*. Age Concern England, London.

Age Concern England (1991). *Older People in the United Kingdom—Some Basic Facts*. Age Concern England, London.

Age Concern Institute of Gerontology (1991). Analysis of data from GHS 1988 supplied via OPCS and ESRC Data Archive, King's College, London. ACIOG, unpublished material. (OPCS bears no responsibility for analysis or interpretation of this data.)

Aldeman, R. *et al.* (1988). A well elderly program: an intergenerational model in medical education. *The Gerontologist*, **28(3)**, 409–13.

Allat, P. (1990). *Women into Retirement: Change and Transition*, seminar paper. Pre-Retirement Association, and the Centre for Retirement Education. Guildford.

Allat, P. *et al.* (Eds) (1987). *Women and the Life Cycle: Transitions and Turning Points*. Macmillan, London.

Allen, I. (1988). Ageing as a feminist issue. *Policy Studies*, **9(2)**, 35–50.

Allen, I. *et al.* (1992). *Elderly People: Choice, Participation and Satisfaction*. Policy Studies Institute, London.

Allen, K. (1989). *Single Women/Family Ties: Life Histories of Older Women*. Sage Publications Inc., Newbury Park, CA.

Arber, S. and Ginn, J. (1991a). Gender, class and income inequalities in later life. *British Journal of Sociology*, **42(3)**, 369–96.

Arber, S. and Ginn, J. (1991b). The invisibility of age: gender and class in later life. *The Sociological Review*, **39(2)**, 260–91.

Arber, S. and Ginn, J. (1991c). *Gender and Later Life—A Sociological Analysis of Resources and Constraints*. Sage Publications Ltd, London.

Argyle, M. and Henderson, M.   (1984).   The rules of friendship. *Journal of Personal and Social Relationships*, **1**, 211–37.

Armstrong, M.J. and Goldsteen, K.S.   (1990).   Friendship support patterns of older American women. *Journal of Aging Studies*, **4(4)**, 391–404.

Askham, J. *et al.*   (1990).   *A Review of Research on Falls among Elderly People*. Department of Trade and Industry, London.

Askham, J. *et al.*   (1992).   *Caring. The Importance of Third Age Carers*, Research Paper no. 6. The Carnegie United Kingdom Trust, Dunfermline.

Atchley, R.C.   (1971).   Retirement and leisure participation: continuity or crisis? *The Gerontologist*, **1(Spring)**, 13–17.

Atkin, K. *et al.*   (1989).   Asian elders' knowledge of community, social and health services. *New Community*, **15(3)**, 439–45.

Audit Commission for England and Wales   (1986).   *Making a Reality of Community Care*. HMSO, London.

Avery, G.   (1991).   *The Best Type of Girl: A History of Girls' Independent Schools*. Andre Deutsch, London.

Barker, J.   (1984a).   Out in the cold. *Nursing Times*, **80(30)**, 19–20.

Barker, J.   (1984b).   *Black and Asian Old People in Britain*. Age Concern England, London.

Barrow, J.   (1982).   West Indian families: an insider's perspective. In *Families in Britain*, Rapoport, R. *et al.* (Eds), pp.220–32. Routledge and Kegan Paul, London.

Bayley, M.   (1973).   *Mental Handicap and Community Care*. Routledge and Kegan Paul, London.

Beddoe, D.   (1989).   *Back to Home and Duty*. Pandora Press, London.

Bedford, V. and Gold, D. (Eds)   (1989).   Siblings in later life: a neglected family relationship. *American Behavioural Scientist* (special issue), **33(1)**, 6–126.

Beechey, V. and Perkins, T.   (1987).   *Women, Part-time Work and the Labour Market*. Polity Press, Cambridge.

Begum, N.   (1991).   *At the Mercy of Others: Disabled Women's Experiences of Receiving Personal Care*, Paper presented to the BSA Annual Conference, Manchester, March.

Bell, A. and Weinberg, M.   (1978).   *Homosexualities: A Study of Diversity Among Men and Women*. Simon & Schuster, New York.

Bengtson, V.   (1989).   The problem of generations: age group contrasts, continuities and social change. In *The Course of Later Life: Research and Reflections*, Bengtson, V. and Schaie, K. (Eds), pp.237–62. Springer Verlag, New York, NY.

Bennett, G.J. and Ebrahim, S.   (1992).   *The Essentials of Health Care of the Elderly*. Edward Arnold, London.

Bennett, G.J. and Kingston, P.   (in press).   *Elder Abuse*. Chapman Hall, London.

Beresford, P. and Croft, S.   (in press).   *Citizen Involvement: A Practical Guide for Change*. Macmillan, London.

Berger Gluck, S. and Patai, D.   (1991).   *Women's Words—The Feminist Practice of Oral History*. Routledge and Kegan Paul, London.

Bernard, J.   (1973).   *The Future of Marriage.* Souvenir Press, London.
Bernard, J.   (1976).   Homosociality and female depression. *Journal of Social Issues*, **32(4)**, 213–38.
Bernard, M.   (1982).   *Leisure Defined: A Review of the Literature*, Occasional Paper no. 3. Dept of Geography, University of Keele, Keele.
Bernard, M.   (1983).   *Leisure-rich and Leisure-poor: The Place of Leisure in the Lifestyles of Young Adults*, Unpublished PhD thesis. University of Keele, Keele.
Bernard, M.   (1984).   Leisure in later life: an introduction to theory and practice. In *Leisure in Later Life*, Bernard, M. (Ed.), pp.1–19. The Beth Johnson Foundation, Stoke-on-Trent.
Bernard, M.   (1985).   *Health Education and Activities for Older People: A Review of Current Practice*, Working Papers on the Health of Older People No. 2. Health Education Council, in association with the Department of Adult Education, University of Keele, Keele.
Bernard, M.   (1988).   Taking charge: strategies for self-empowered health behaviour amongst older people. *Health Education Journal*, **47(2/3)**, 87–90.
Bernard, M.   (1989).   Research in action: self-health care and older people. *Hygie-International Journal of Health Education*, **8(2)**, 11–15.
Bernard, M.   (1990).   *Beyond Our Present Imagination: Leisure and Lifestyle in Later Life.* Centre for Policy on Ageing, London.
Bernard, M. and Ivers, V.   (1986).   Peer health counselling: a way of countering dependency? In *Dependency and Interdependency in Old Age: Theoretical Perspectives and Policy Alternatives*, Phillipson, C. et al. (Eds), pp.288–99. Croom Helm, London.
Bernard, M. and Phillipson, C.   (1991).   Self-care and health in old age. In *Nursing Elderly People*, second edition, Redfern, S. (Ed.), pp.405–15. Churchill Livingstone, Edinburgh.
Berry, S. et al.   (1981).   *Report on a Survey of West Indian Pensioners in Nottingham*, mimeo. Nottingham Social Services Department, Nottingham.
Beuret, K.   (1991).   Women and transport. In *Women's Issues in Social Policy*, Maclean, M. and Groves, D. (Eds), pp. 61–75. Routledge, London.
Beveridge, Sir W.   (1942).   *Social Insurance and Allied Services*, Cmd 6406. HMSO, London.
Bhalla, A. and Blakemore K.   (1981).   *Elders of the Ethnic Minority Groups.* All Faiths For One Race, Birmingham.
Binstock, R.H.   (1985).   The oldest old: a fresh perspective, or compassionate ageism revisited. *Milbank Memory Fund Quarterly*, **63(2)**, 420–51.
Blacher, M.   (1983).   Elderly vagrants. In *Ageing in Modern Society*, Jerrome, D. (Ed.), pp.61–80. Croom Helm, London.
Blakemore, K.   (1982) Health and illness among the elderly of minority ethnic groups living in Birmingham: some new findings. *Health Trends*, **14**, 69–72.
Blakemore, K.   (1983a).   Ethnicity, self-reported illness and use of

medical services by the elderly. *Postgraduate Medical Journal*, **59**, 668–70.

Blakemore, K. (1983b). Ageing in the inner cities: a comparison of old blacks and whites. In *Ageing in Modern Society*, Jerrome, D. (Ed.), pp.81–103. Croom Helm, London.

Blau, Z. (1973). *Old Age in a Changing Society*. Franklin Watts, New York, NY.

Blaxter, M. (1980). *The Meaning of Disability*, Heinemann Educational, Oxford.

Blaxter, M. (1990). *Health and Lifestyles*. Routledge, London.

Blaxter, M. and Patterson, E. (1982). *Mothers and Daughters: A Three-generational Study of Health, Attitudes and Behaviour*. Heinemann Educational, Oxford.

Block, M. *et al.* (1981). *Women Over Forty*. Springer Verlag, New York, NY.

Bond, J. and Coleman, P. (Eds) (1990). *Ageing in Society—An Introduction to Social Gerontology*. Sage Publications Ltd, London.

Bond, J. *et al.* (1990). The study of ageing. In *Ageing in Society—An Introduction to Social Gerontology*, Bond, J. and Coleman, P. (Eds), pp.17–47. Sage Publications Ltd, London.

Booth, T. (1985). *Home Truths: Old People's Homes and the Outcome of Care*. Gower Publishing Group Ltd, Aldershot.

Bornat, J. (1989). Oral history as a social movement: reminiscence and older people. *Oral History*, **17(2)**, 16–24.

Bornat, J. *et al.* (1985). *A Manifesto For Old Age*. Pluto Press, London.

Bould, M. (1990). Trapped within four walls. *Community Care*, **19(April)**, 17–19.

Boys, J. *et al.* (1984). House design and women's roles. In *Making Space: Women and the Man Made Environment*, Matrix (Eds), pp.55–80. Pluto Press, London.

Braybon, G. and Summerfield, P. (1987). *Out of the Cage: Women's Experiences in Two World Wars*. Pandora Press, London.

Brayne, C. and Ames, D. (1988). The epidemiology of mental disorders in old age. In *Mental Health Problems in Old Age*, Gearing, B. *et al.* (Eds), pp.10–26. John Wiley and Sons Ltd, Chichester.

Brehm, H.P. (1968). Sociology and aging: orientation and research. *The Gerontologist*, **8(1)**, 24–32.

Briggs, A. and Oliver, J. (Eds) (1985). *Caring: Experiences of Looking After Disabled Relatives*. Routledge and Kegan Paul, London.

Brion, M. and Tinker, A. (1980). *Women in Housing: Access and Influence*. Housing Centre Trust, London.

Brody, E. (1981). 'Women in the middle' and family help to older people. *The Gerontologist*, **21(5)**, 471–80.

Bromley, D.B. (1974). *The Psychology of Human Ageing*. Penguin, Harmondsworth.

Brown, C. (1984). *Black and White Britain*. William Heinemann, London.

Brown, G. and Harris, T. (1978). *The Social Origins of Depression*. Tavistock, London.

Brubaker, T.H. (1985). *Later Life Families*. Sage Publications Inc., Newbury Park, CA.

Bryan, B. *et al.* (1985). *The Heart of the Race: Black Women's Lives in Britain*. Virago Press, London.

Buhler, C. (1935). *From Birth To Maturity*. Routledge and Kegan Paul, London.

Bull, J. and Poole, L. (1989). *Not Rich, Not Poor: A Study of Housing Options for Elderly People on Middle Incomes*. SHAC and Anchor Housing Trust, London.

Burns, B. and Phillipson, C. (1986). *Drugs, Ageing and Society: Social and Pharmacological Perspectives*. Croom Helm, London.

Burnside, I. (1985). Adjustment to family losses; grief in frail elderly women. In *The Physical and Mental Health of Aged Women*, Haug, M. *et al.* (Eds), pp.152–65. Springer Verlag, New York.

Bury, M. (1988). Arguments about ageing: long life and its consequences. In *The Ageing Population: Burden or Challenge?*, Wells, N. and Freer, C. (Eds), pp.17–31. Macmillan, London.

Bury, M. and Holme, A. (1991). *Life After Ninety*. Routledge, London.

Caesar, G. (1987). *Black Women Talk: The Experience of Elderly Black Women of Caribbean Origin in Britain*, dissertation, B.A. Applied Social Studies. Polytechnic of North London, London.

Campbell, B. (1987). *The Iron Ladies: Why Do Women Vote Tory?* Virago Press, London.

Cant, B. and Hemmings, S. (Eds) (1988). *Radical Records: Thirty Years of Lesbian and Gay History 1957–87*. Routledge, London.

Caplan, P. (Ed.) (1987). *The Cultural Construction of Sexuality*. Tavistock, London.

Carter, A. and Nash, C. (in press). *Pensioners Forums*. Pre-Retirement Association and Centre for Health and Retirement Education, Guildford.

Central Statistical Office (1989). *Social Trends 19*. HMSO, London.

Central Statistical Office (1990). *Social Trends 20*. HMSO, London.

Central Statistical Office (1991). *Social Trends 21*. HMSO, London.

Centre for Policy on Ageing (1984). *Home Life: A Code of Practice for Residential Care*. CPA, London.

Centre for Policy on Ageing (1990). *Community Life: A Code of Practice for Community Care*. CPA, London.

Centre for Policy on Ageing (1992). *Leisure Life: A Local Authority Code of Practice for the Effective Provision of Leisure to Older People*. CPA/Help the Aged/Age Concern/Chief Leisure Officers Association, London.

Charlesworth, A. *et al.* (1984). *Carers and Services: A Comparison of Men and Women Caring for Dependent Elderly People*. Equal Opportunities Commission, Manchester.

Chodorow, N. (1978). *The Reproduction of Mothering*. United California Press, CA.

Clark, M. (1969). Cultural values and dependency in later life. In *The Dependency of Old People*, Kalish, R. (Ed.), pp.59–72. University of Michigan Press, Ann Arbor, MI.

Clarke, J. and Critcher, C. (1985). *The Devil Makes Work: Leisure in Capitalist Britain*. Macmillan, London.

Clennell, S. (1987). *Older Students in Adult Education*. Open University, Milton Keynes.

Clennell, S. (Ed.) (1990). *Older Students in Europe*. Open University, Milton Keynes.

Cockerham, W.C. *et al.* (1983). Aging and perceived health status. *Journal of Gerontology*, **38**, 349–55.

Cohen, C.I. (1989). Social ties and the friendship patterns of old, homeless men. In *Older Adult Friendships*, Adams, R.G. and Blieszner, R. (Eds), pp.222–42. Sage Publications Inc., Newbury Park, CA.

Coleman, P. (1986). *The Ageing Process and the Role of Reminiscence*. John Wiley, London.

Coleman, P. (1990a). Psychological ageing. In *Ageing in Society—An Introduction to Social Gerontology*, Bond, J. and Coleman, P. (Eds), pp.62–88. Sage Publications Ltd, London.

Coleman, P. (1990b). Adjustment in later life. In *Ageing in Society— An Introduction to Social Gerontology*, Bond, J. and Coleman, P. (Eds), pp.89–122. Sage Publications Ltd, London.

Coleman, P. and MacCulloch, A. (1985). The study of psychological change in adult life. In *Lifespan and Change in a Gerontological Perspective*, Munnichs J. *et al.*, pp.239–55. Academic Press, San Diego, CA.

Cooperstock, R. (1978). Sex differences in psychotropic drug use. *Social Science and Medicine*, **12b**, 179–86.

Coote, A. and Campbell, B. (1982). *Sweet Freedom*. Picador, London.

Copeland, J.R.M. *et al.* (1987). Range of mental illness among the elderly in the community. *British Journal of Psychiatry*, **150**, 815–23.

Coppard, L.C. *et al.* (1984). *Self-health Care and Older People—A Manual for Public Policy and Programme Development*. World Health Organization, Copenhagen.

Copper, B. (1988). *Over The Hill, Reflections on Ageism Between Women*. The Crossing Press, Freedom, CA.

Cornwell, J. (1984). *Hard Earned Lives: Accounts of Health and Illness from East London*. Tavistock, London.

Cornwell, J. (1989). *The Consumers' View: Elderly People and Community Health Services*. King's Fund Centre, London.

Cox, B.D. *et al.* (1987). *The Health and Lifestyles Survey*. The Health Promotion Research Trust, London.

Crowley, H. and Himmelweit, S. (1992). *Knowing Women—Feminism and Knowledge*. Polity Press in Association with the Open University, Cambridge.

Cumming, E. and Henry, W.E. (1961). *Growing Old: the Process of Disengagement*. Basic Books, New York.

Cunningham-Burley, S. (1985). Constructing grandparenthood. *Sociology*, **19(3)**, 421–36.

Curtis, Z. (1989). Older women and feminism: don't say sorry. *Feminist Review*, **31(Spring)**, 143–7.

Dale, A. *et al.* (1987). The household structure of the elderly in Britain. *Ageing and Society*, **7(1)**, 37–56.

Dalley, G. (1988). *Ideologies of Caring: Rethinking Community and Collectivism*. Macmillan Educational Ltd, Houndmills.

Dalley, G. (Ed.) (1991). *Disability and Social Policy*. Policy Studies Institute, London.

Dant, T. *et al.* (1989). *Co-ordinating Care. The Final Report of the Care for Elderly People at Home (CEPH) Project, Gloucester*, for the Department of Health and Social Welfare, The Open University. Policy Studies Institute, London.

Davidoff, L. *et al.* (1976). Landscape with figures: home and community in English society. In *The Rights and Wrongs of Women*, Mitchell, J. and Oakley, A. (Eds), pp.139–75. Penguin, Harmondsworth.

Davidson, F. (1990). Occupational pensions and equal treatment. *Journal of Social Welfare Law*, 5, 310–31.

Davies, B. and Ward, S. (1992). *Women and Personal Pensions*. Equal Opportunities Commission/HMSO, London.

Dean, K. (1982). Self-care: what people do for themselves. In *Self-help and Health in Europe—New Approaches in Health Care*, Hatch, S. and Kickbusch, I. (Eds), pp.20–31. World Health Organization, Copenhagen.

Dean, K. *et al.* (1986). *Self-care and Health in Old Age*. Croom Helm, London.

Decalmer, P. and Glendenning, F.G. (Eds) (in press). *The Mistreatment of Elderly People*. Sage Publications Ltd, London.

de Carlo, T.J. (1974). Recreation participation and successful aging. *Journal of Gerontology*, 29(4), 416–22.

Deem, R. (1986). *All Work and No Play?—The Sociology of Women and Leisure*. Open University Press, Milton Keynes.

Department of Employment (1989). *Labour Force Survey 1987*. HMSO, London.

Department of Employment (1990). *New Earnings Survey*. HMSO, London.

Department of the Environment (1983). *English House Condition Survey, 1981, Part 1*. HMSO, London.

Department of the Environment (1988). *English House Condition Survey, 1986*. HMSO, London.

Department of Health (1988). *Caring for People*. HMSO, London.

Department of Health (1991). *Survey of Age, Sex and Length of Stay Characteristics of Residents of Homes for Elderly People and Younger People Who are Physically Handicapped in England at 31st March 1988, Personal Social Services, Local Authority Statistics*. HMSO, London.

Department of Health and Social Security (1971). *Better Services for the Mentally Handicapped*, Cmnd. 4683. HMSO, London.

Department of Health and Social Security (1975). *Better Services for the Mentally Ill*, Cmnd. 6233. HMSO, London.

Department of Health and Social Security (1976). *Priorities for Health and Personal Social Services in England*. HMSO, London.

Department of Health and Social Security (1978). *A Happier Old Age*. HMSO, London.

Department of Health and Social Security (1981). *Growing Older*, Cmnd. 8173. HMSO, London.

Department of Health and Social Security (1984). *Population, Pension Costs and Pensioners' Incomes: Background Paper for the Inquiry into Provision for Retirement*. HMSO, London.

Department of Health and Social Security (1987). *Hospital In-Patient Enquiry, 1985*, Series MB4, No. 27. HMSO, London.

Department of Health and Social Security (1989). *Mental Health Statistics for England 1986*. HMSO, London.

Department of Social Security (1991a). *Options for Equality in State Pension Age*. HMSO, London.

Department of Social Security (1991b). *Social Security Statistics 1990*. HMSO, London.

Dex, S. and Phillipson, C. (1986). Older women in the labour market: a review of current trends. *Critical Social Policy*, **15**, 79–83.

Dixey, R. (1987). 'Eyes down': a study of bingo. In *Relative Freedoms: Women and Leisure*, Wimbush, E. and Talbot, M. (Eds), pp.91–101. Open University Press, Milton Keynes.

Dixey, R. and Talbot, M. (1982). *Women, Leisure and Bingo*. Trinity and All Saints College, Leeds.

Dobbin, I. (1980). *Leisure and the Elderly*. Centre for Leisure Studies, University of Salford, Salford.

Donaldson, L.J. and Odell, A. (1984). *Aspects of Health and Social Needs of Elderly Asians in Leicester: A Community Survey*. Department of Community Medicine, Leicester.

Donovan, J. (1986). *We Don't Buy Sickness It Just Comes*. Gower Publishing Group Ltd, Aldershot.

Douglas, J. (1992). Black women's health matters: putting black women on the research agenda. In *Women's Health Matters*, Roberts, H. (Ed.), pp.33–46. Routledge, London.

Dowd, J.J. (1980). *Stratification Among the Aged*. Brooks/Cole, Monterey, CA.

Dower, M. *et al.* (1979). *Leisure Provision and People's Needs. Report for the Department of the Environment by the Institute of Family and Environmental Research and Dartington Amenity Research Trust.* HMSO, London.

Duncan, D. (1991). Communication. In *Multicultural Health Care and Rehabilitation*, Squires, A. (Ed.), pp.78–85. Edward Arnold and Age Concern England, London.

Dunker, B. (1987). Aging lesbians. In *Lesbian Psychologies*, Boston Lesbian Psychologies Collective (Eds), pp.72–82. University of Illinois Press, Champaign IL.

Eastman, M. (1984). *Old Age Abuse*. Age Concern England, London.

Ebrahim, S. (1992). Health of elderly Asian women. In *Health Care for Older Women*, George, J. and Ebrahim, S. (Eds), pp.168–78. Oxford University Press, Oxford.

Ehrenreich, and English, D. (1979). *For Her Own Good: Fifty Years of the Experts' Advice to Women*. Pluto Press, London.

Eichenbaum, L. and Orbach, S. (1985). *Understanding Women*. Penguin, London.

Eisenstein, H. (1984). *Contemporary Feminist Thought*. Unwin, London.

Ellis, B. (1989). *Pensions in Britain 1955–1975*. HMSO, London.

Engels, F. (1884). *The Origins of the Family, Private Property and the State*, republished in 1985. Penguin, Harmondsworth.

Equal Opportunities Commission (1980). *The Experience of Caring for*

Elderly and Handicapped Dependants: Survey Report. EOC, Manchester.

Equal Opportunities Commission (1982a). *Caring for the Elderly and Handicapped*. EOC, Manchester.

Equal Opportunities Commission (1982b). *Who Cares for the Carers*. EOC, Manchester.

Equal Opportunities Commission (1989). Age discrimination: over the hill at 45? *Equal Opportunities Review*, **25(May/June)**.

Erikson, E.H. (1950). *Childhood and Society*. Hogarth Press, London.

Erikson, E.H. *et al.* (1986). *Vital Involvement in Old Age: the Experience of Old Age in Our Time*. Norton, New York, NY.

Eurolink Age (1985). *The Situation of Older Women in Europe—Report of Seminar*. Eurolink Age, Luxembourg.

Evandrou, M. (1987). *The Use of Domiciliary Services by the Elderly: A Survey*. Suntory-Toyota International Centre for Economics and Related Disciplines, London School of Economics, London.

Evandrou, M. (1990). *Challenging the Invisibility of Carers: Mapping Informal Care Nationally*. Suntory-Toyota International Centre for Economics and Related Disciplines, London School of Economics, London.

Evers, H. (1983). Elderly women and disadvantage. In *Ageing in Modern Society*, Jerrome D. (Ed.), pp.25–44. Croom Helm, London.

Evers, H. (1985). The frail elderly woman: emergent questions in ageing and women's health. In *Women, Health and Healing: Towards a New Perspective*, Lewin, E. and Oleson, V. (Eds), pp.86–112. Tavistock, London.

Falkingham, J. and Victor, C. (1991). *The Myth of the Woopie? Incomes, the Elderly, and Targeting Welfare*, Discussion Paper WSP/55, The Welfare State Programme, STICERD. London School of Economics, London.

Family Policy Studies Centre (1991). *An Ageing Population, FactSheet 2*. Family Policy Studies Centre, London.

Farrah, M. (1986). *Black Elders in Leicester: An Action Research Report on the Needs of Black Elderly People of African Descent from the Caribbean*, mimeo. Social Services Department, Leicestershire County Council, Leicester.

Featherstone, M. (1987). Leisure, symbolic power and the life course. In *Sport, Leisure and Social Relations. Sociological Review Monograph No. 33*, Horne, J. *et al.* (Eds), pp.113–38. Routledge, London.

Featherstone, M. and Hepworth, M. (1989). Ageing and old age: reflections on the postmodern life course. In *Becoming and Being Old*, B. Bytheway *et al.* (Eds), pp.143–57. Sage Publications Ltd, London.

Fennell, G. (1986). *Anchor's Older People: What Do They Think?* Anchor Housing Association, Oxford.

Fennell, G. *et al.* (1988). *The Sociology of Old Age*. Open University Press, Milton Keynes.

Fenton, C.S. (1986). *Race, Health and Welfare. Afro-Caribbeans and South Asian People in Central Bristol—Health and Social Services*. Department of Sociology, University of Bristol, Bristol.

Fenton, C.S.   (1987).   *Ageing Minorities*. Commission for Racial
    Equality, London.
Fenton, C.S.   (1988).   Health, work and growing old: the
    Afro-Caribbean experience. *New Community*, **15(3)**, 426–43.
Fenton, C.S.   (1991).   Ethnic minority populations in Britain. In
    Multicultural Health Care and Rehabilitation, Squires, A. (Ed.),
    pp.3–16. Edward Arnold and Age Concern England, London.
Ferraro, K.F.   (1987).   Double jeopardy to health for black older adults?
    Journal of Gerontology, **42(5)**, 538–53.
Finch, J.   (1984).   Community care: developing non-sexist alternatives.
    Critical Social Policy, **9(3/3)**, 6–18.
Finch, J.   (1989).   *Family Obligations and Social Change*. Polity Press,
    Cambridge.
Finch, J.   (1990).   Filial obligations and kin support for elderly people.
    Ageing and Society, **10(2)**, 151–75.
Finch, J. and Groves, D.   (1980).   Community care and the family: a case
    for equal opportunities. *Journal of Social Policy*, **9(4)**, 487–511.
Finch, J. and Groves, D.   (1982).   By women for women: caring for the
    frail elderly. *Women's Studies International Forum*, **5(5)**, 427–38.
Finch, J. and Groves, D. (Eds)   (1983).   *A Labour of Love: Women,
    Work and Caring*. Routledge and Kegan Paul, London.
Finch, J. and Groves, D.   (1985).   Old girl, old boy: gender divisions in
    social work with the elderly. In *Women, the Family and Social Work*,
    Brook, E. and Davis, A. (Eds), pp.92–111. Tavistock, London.
Fiske, M. and Chiriboga, D.   (1985).   The interweaving of societal and
    personal change in adulthood. In *Life-Span and Change in a
    Gerontological Perspective*, Munnichs, J.M.A. *et al.* (Eds), pp.177–
    209. Academic Press Inc., San Diego, CA.
Fleiss, A.   (1985).   *Home Ownership Alternatives for The Elderly*.
    HMSO, London.
Fletcher, A.   (1992).   Controversies in screening for breast and cervical
    cancer. In *Health Care for Older Women*, George, J. and Ebrahim, S.
    (Eds), pp.222–35. Oxford University Press, Oxford.
Fogarty, M. *et al.*   (1980).   *Women in Top Jobs 1968–1979*. Heinemann,
    London.
Fooken, I.   (1985).   Old and female: psychosocial concomitants of the
    aging process in a group of older women. In *Life-Span and Change
    in a Gerontological Perspective*, Munnichs, J.M.A. *et al.* (Eds), pp.77–
    101. Academic Press Inc., San Diego, CA.
Ford, J. and Sinclair, R.   (1987).   *Sixty Years On: Women Talk About
    Old Age*. Women's Press, London.
Forster, M.   (1989).   *Have the Men had Enough?* Penguin,
    Harmondsworth.
Francis, D.   (1990).   The significance of work friends in late life. *Journal
    of Ageing Studies*, **4(4)**, 405–24.
Franks, H.   (1987).   *What Every Woman Should Know About Retirement*.
    Age Concern England, London.
Franz, C. and White, K.   (1985).   Individuation and attachment in
    personality development: extending Erikson's theory. *Journal of
    Personality*, **53**, 224–56.

Freer, C.B. (1985). Geriatric screening: a reappraisal of the preventive strategies in the care of the elderly. *Journal of the Royal College of General Practitioners*, **35**, 288–90.

Fries, J.F. (1980) Ageing, natural death and the compression of morbidity. *New England Journal of Medicine*, **303(3)**, 130–35.

Fries, J.F. (1989). Reduction of the national morbidity. In *Aging and Health*, Lewis, S. (Ed.), pp.3–22. Lewis, MI.

Froggatt, A. (1985). Listening to the voices of older women; creativity and social work responses. In *Ageing—Recent Advances and Responses*, Butler, A. (Ed.), pp.35–50. Croom Helm, London.

Fry, V. *et al.* (1990). *Pensioners and the Public Purse*, IFS Report Series 36. Institute for Fiscal Studies, London.

Fryer, P. (1984). Staying Power: The History of Black People in Britain. Pluto Press, London.

Garner, J.D. and Mercer, S.O. (Eds) (1989). *Women As They Age: Challenge, Opportunity and Triumph*. Haworth Press, New York.

Gaylord, S. (1989). Women and aging: A psychological perspective. In *Women As They Age: Challenge, Opportunity and Triumph*, Garner, J.D. and Mercer, S.O. (Eds), pp.69–93. Haworth Press, New York.

Gee, E.M. and Kimball, M.M. (1987). *Women and Aging*. Butterworths, Toronto.

George, J. and Ebrahim, S. (Eds) (1992). *Health Care for Older Women*. Oxford University Press, Oxford.

Gibb, K. *The Times*, 28.6.90.

Gibson, C. (1990). Widowhood: patterns, problems and choices. In *Aspects of Ageing, Social Policy Papers No. 3*, Bury, M. and Macnicol, J. (Eds), pp.82–103. Department of Social Policy and Social Science, Royal Holloway and Bedford New College, London.

Gibson, M.J. (1985). *Older Women Around the World*. International Federation on Aging, Washington DC.

Gilligan, C. (1982). *In A Different Voice*. Harvard University Press, Cambridge, MA.

Glendenning, F. (1983). Ethnic minority elderly people. In *Social Work and Ethnicity*, Cheetham, J. (Ed.), pp.122–32. Harper and Row, London.

Glendenning, F. and Pearson, M. (1988). *Black and Ethnic Minority Elders in Britain:. Health Needs and Access to Services*, Working Papers on the Health of Older People, No. 6. Health Education Authority in association with the Centre for Social Gerontology, University of Keele, Keele.

Glendinning, C. (1992). *The Costs of Informal Caring*. HMSO, London.

Glendinning, C. and Millar, J. (Eds) (1987). *Women and Poverty in Britain*. Wheatsheaf, Brighton.

Glendinning, C. and Millar, J. (1991). Poverty and the forgotten Englishwoman. In *Women's Issues in Social Policy*, Maclean, M. and Groves, D. (Eds), pp.20–37. Routledge, London.

Godlove, C. *et al.* (1982). *Time for Action: An Observation Study of Elderly People in Four Different Care Environments*. Joint Unit for Social Services, University of Sheffield, Sheffield.

Golant, S. (1982). Individual differences underlying the dwelling

satisfaction of the elderly. *Journal of Social Issues*, **38(3)**, 121–38.
Goldsmith, S. (1974). *Mobility Housing*. Department of the Environment, London.
Gove, W. (1984). Gender differences in mental and physical illness: the effects of fixed roles and nurturant roles. *Social Science and Medicine*, **19**, 77–91.
Gove, W. and Hughes, M. (1979). Possible causes of the apparent sex differences in physical health: an empirical investigation. *American Sociological Review*, **44**, 126–46.
Graham, H. (1983). Caring: a labour of love. In *A Labour of Love: Women, Work and Caring*, Finch, J. and Groves, D. (Eds), pp.13–30. Routledge and Kegan Paul, London.
Grant, G. (1990). Elderly parents with handicapped children. *Journal of Aging Studies*, **4(4)**, 359–74.
Grant, V. (1986). *Day Centres for the Elderly*. Benton Ross, Auckland.
Greater London Council Women's Committee (1985). *Women on the Move: GLC Survey on Women and Transport*, no. 3. GLC, London.
Green, D. (1992). Liberty, poverty and the underclass: a classical-liberal approach to public policy. In *Understanding the Underclass*, Smith, D.J. (Ed.), pp.68–87. PSI, London.
Green, E. *et al.* (1990). *Women's Leisure—What Leisure?* Macmillan, London.
Green, H. (1988). *Informal Carers*, OPCS Series GHS, No. 15, Supplement A. HMSO, London.
Greer, G. (1991). *The Change—Women, Ageing and the Menopause*. Hamish Hamilton Limited, London.
Griffiths, Sir R. (1988). *Community Care: Agenda for Action*. HMSO, London.
Groombridge, B. (1980). Education, outreach and the media. In *Outreach Education and the Elders: Theory and Practice*, Glendenning, F. (Ed.), pp.9–22. The Beth Johnson Foundation in association with the Department of Adult Education, University of Keele, Stoke-on-Trent.
Groves, D. (1983). Members and survivors: women and retirement pensions legislation. In *Women's Welfare, Women's Rights*, Lewis, J. (Ed.), pp.38–63. Croom Helm, London.
Groves, D. (1987). Occupational pension provision and women's poverty in old age. In *Women and Poverty in Britain*, Glendinning, C. and Millar, J. (Eds), pp.199–217. Wheatsheaf, Brighton.
Groves, D. (1991). Women and financial provision for old age. In *Women's Issues in Social Policy*, Maclean, M. and Groves D. (Eds), pp.38–60. Routledge, London.
Grundy, E. (1983). Demography and old age. *Journal of the American Geriatrics Society*, **31(6)**, 325–32.
The Guardian Newspaper, 27.6.91.
Gutmann, D.L. (1987). *Reclaimed Powers: Towards a New Psychology of Men and Women in Later Life*. Basic Books, New York.
Hagestad, G. (1985a). Older women in intergenerational relations. In *The Physical and Mental Health of Aged Women*, Haug, M., *et al.* (Eds), pp.137–51. Springer Verlag, New York.

References 209

Hagestad, G. (1985b). Continuity and connectedness. In *Grandparenthood*, Bengtson, V. and Robertson, J. (Eds), pp.31–48. Sage Publications Inc., Newbury Park, CA.

Hall, S. (1985). Letter. *Spare Rib*, **154(May)**, 20.

Hall Carpenter Archives Lesbian Oral History Group (1989). *Inventing Ourselves: Lesbian Life Stories*. Routledge, London.

Hand, J. (1983). Shopping-bag women: aging deviants in the city. In *Older Women: Issues and Prospects*, Markson, E. (Ed.), pp.155–78.. Lexington Books, Lexington, MA.

Hansard (30 October 1986). *House of Commons Debates, 1985–86*. Vol. 103, cols 231–4, 734–5.

Hardman, A. (1992). Exercise and older women. In *Health Care for Older Women*, George, J. and Ebrahim, S. (Eds), pp.222–35. Oxford University Press, Oxford.

Harrop, A. (1990). *The Employment Position of Older Women in Europe*. Age Concern Institute of Gerontology, King's College, London.

Hart, N. (1976). *When Marriage Ends*. Tavistock, London.

Haskey, J. (1990). The ethnic minority population of Great Britain; estimates by ethnic group and country of birth. *Population Trends*, **60**, 35–8.

Havighurst, R.J. (1953). *Human Development and Education*. Longman Group UK Ltd, Harlow.

Havighurst, R.J. (1963). Successful aging. In *Processes of Aging*, Vol. 1, Williams, R.H. *et al.* (Eds), pp.299–320. Atherton, New York, NY.

Heinemann, G. and Evans, P. (1990). Widowhood: loss, change and adaptation. In *Family Relationships in Later Life*, second edition, Brubaker, T. (Ed.), pp.142–68. Sage Publications Inc., Newbury Park, CA.

Hemer, J. and Stanyer, A. (1986). *Survival Guides for Widows*. Age Concern England, London.

Hemmings, S. (1985). *A Wealth of Experience: The Lives of Older Women*. Pandora Press, London.

Henderson, K.A. (1990). The meaning of leisure for women: an integrative review of the research. *Journal of Leisure Research*, **22(3)**, 228–43.

Henderson, K.A. *et al.* (1989). *A Leisure of One's Own: A Feminist Perspective on Women's Leisure*. Venture Publishing Inc., Philadelphia, PA.

Hendricks, J. and Hendricks, C.D. (1977). *Aging in Mass Society*. Winthrop, Cambridge, MA.

Henwood, M. (1990a). *Community Care and Elderly People—Policy, Practice, and Research Review*. Family Policy Studies Centre, London.

Henwood, M. (1990b). No sense of urgency. In *Age: The Unrecognized Discrimination*, McEwen, E. (Ed.), pp.43–57. Age Concern England, London.

Hess, B. (1979). Sex roles, friendship and the life course. *Research on Aging*, **1(4)**, 494–515.

Hess, B. and Soldo, B. (1985). Husband and wife networks. In *Social*

Support Networks and Care of the Elderly, Sauer, W. and Coward, R. (Eds), pp.69–92. Springer Verlag, New York, NY.

Hicks, C. (1988). *Who Cares? Looking After People at Home*. Virago Press, London.

Himmelfarb, S. (1984). Age and sex differences in the mental health of older persons. *Journal of Consulting and Clinical Psychology*, **52(5)**, 844–56.

Holland, B. and Levando-Hundt, G. (1987). *Coventry Ethnic Minorities Elderly Survey: Method, Data and Applied Action*. Ethnic Minorities Development Unit, City of Coventry, Coventry.

Howell, S.C. (1983). The meaning of place in old age. In *Aging and Milieu: Environmental Perspectives on Growing Old*, Rowles, G.R. and Ohta, R.J. (Eds), pp.97–107. Academic Press Inc., San Diego, CA.

Hughes, B. (1990). Quality of life. In *Researching Social Gerontology*. Peace, S.M. (Ed.), pp.46–58. Sage Publications Ltd, London.

Hume, C. (1991). Occupational therapy with ethnic minority clients. In *Multicultural Health Care and Rehabilitation*, Squires, A. (Ed.), pp.133–42. Edward Arnold and Age Concern England, London.

Hunt, A. (1968). *A Survey of Women's Employment*. HMSO, London.

Hunt, A. (1978). *The Elderly at Home—A Study of People Aged 65 and Over Living in the Community in 1976*. HMSO, London.

Hunt, A. (1988). Women and paid work: issues of inequality: an overview. In *Women and Paid Work*, Hunt, A. (Ed.), pp.1–22. Macmillan, London.

Huyck, M.H. (1977). Sex and the older woman. In *Looking Ahead: A Woman's Guide to the Problems and Joys of Growing Older*, Troll, L. *et al.* (Eds). Prentice Hall, Englewood Cliffs, NJ.

Huyck, M.H. (1989). Midlife parental imperatives. In *Midlife Loss: Coping Strategies*, Kalish, R. (Ed.), pp.115–48. Sage Publications Inc., Newbury Park, CA.

Itzin, C. and Phillipson, C. (in press). *Breaking Down Age Barriers in Employment*. Metropolitan Training and Recruitment Agency (METRA), Solihull.

✓ Ivers, V. (1984). Development of leisure opportunities in North Staffordshire. In *Leisure in Later Life: Examples of Community Based Initiatives*, Bernard, M. (Ed.), pp.55–64. The Beth Johnson Foundation, Stoke-on-Trent.

✓ Ivers, V. and Meade, K. (1991). *Older Volunteers and Peer Health Counselling: A New Approach to Training and Development*. The Beth Johnson Foundation, Stoke-on-Trent.

Jefferys, M. and Thane, P. (1989). Introduction: an ageing society and ageing people. In *Growing Old in the Twentieth Century*, Jefferys, M. (Ed.), pp.1–18. Routledge, London.

Jerrome, D.M. (1981). The significance of friendship for women in later life. *Ageing and Society*, **1(2)**, 175–97.

Jerrome, D.M. (1983). Lonely women in a friendship club. *British Journal of Guidance and Counselling*, **11(1)**, 10–20.

Jerrome, D.M. (1988a). Age relations in an English church. *Sociological Review*, **37(4)**, 761–84.

Jerrome, D.M.   (1988b).   That's what it's all about: old people's organizations as a context for ageing. *Journal of Aging Studies*, **2(1)**, 71–81.

Jerrome, D.M.   (1989).   Virtue and vicissitude: a study of the social construction of old age in selected old age organizations. In *Growing Old in the Twentieth Century*, Jefferys, M. (Ed.), pp.151–65. Routledge, London.

Jerrome, D.M.   (1990a).   *Young Wives and Old Widows: Personal and Social Change in the Context of an English Church*, paper to C-SAL Conference. University of Sussex, Brighton.

Jerrome, D.M.   (1990b).   Intimate relationships. In *Ageing in Society— An Introduction to Social Gerontology*, Bond, J. and Coleman, P. (Eds), pp.181–208. Sage Publications Ltd, London.

Jerrome, D.M.   (1990c).   Frailty and friendship. *Journal of Cross-cultural Gerontology*, **5(1)**, 51–64.

Jerrome, D.M.   (1991).   Loneliness: possibilities for intervention. *Journal of Aging Studies*, **5(2)**, 195–208.

Jewish Women in London Group   (1989).   *Generations of Memories: The Voices of Jewish Women*. Women's Press, London.

Jimack, M.   (1983).   *Jewish Senior Citizens in South London: A Study of Social and Community Needs*. Central Council for Jewish Social Service, London.

Johnson, F. and Aries, E.   (1983).   The talk of women friends. *Women's Studies International Forum*, **6(4)**, 351–61.

Johnson, M.L.   (1978).   That was your life: a biographical approach to later life. In *An Ageing Population*, Carver, V. and Liddiard, P. (Eds), pp.99–113. Hodder & Stoughton, Sevenoaks.

Johnson, M.L.   (1989).   *From Generation to Generation: Conflict of the Old, the Young and the State*, Annual Centre for Policy on Ageing/ Niccol Lecture. Centre for Policy on Ageing, London.

Johnson, P. *et al.*   (1989).   *Workers Versus Pensioners: Inter-generational Justice in an Ageing World*. Manchester University Press in association with the Centre for Economic Policy Research, Manchester.

Johnston, S. and Phillipson, C.   (1983).   Education and the older learner: current developments and initiatives. In *Older Learners: The Challenge to Adult Education*, Johnston, S. and Phillipson, C. (eds). Bedford Square Press for Help the Aged, London.

Jones, D.   (1992).   Informal care and community care. In *Health Care for Older Women*, George J. and Ebrahim, S. (Eds), pp.16–26. Oxford University Press, Oxford.

Jones, K.   (1972).   *A History of the Mental Health Services*. Routledge and Kegan Paul, London.

Jorm, A.F. *et al.*   (1987).   The prevalence of dementia: a quantitative integration of the literature. *Acta Psychiatrica Scandinavica*, **76**, 465–79.

Joseph, K. and Sumption, J.   (1979).   *Equality*. John Murray (Publishers) Ltd, London.

Joshi, H.   (1987).   The cost of caring. In *Women and Poverty in Britain*, Glendenning, C. and Millar, J. (Eds), pp.112–33. Wheatsheaf, Brighton.

Joshi, H. (1989). The changing form of women's economic dependency. In *The Changing Population of Britain*, Joshi, H. (Ed.), pp.157–76. Basil Blackwell, Oxford.

Joshi, H. (1990). Changing roles of women in the British labour market and the family. In *Frontiers of Economic Research*, Proceedings of Section F of the British Association for the Advancement of British Science, Oxford, pp.102–28. Macmillan, Basingstoke.

Kart, C.S. (1987). Review essay: the end of conventional gerontology? *Sociology of Health and Illness*, **9(1)**, 76–87.

Keith, L. (1990). The caring partnership. *Community Care*, inside supplement, **22(February)**, v–vi.

Kellaher, L. *et al.* (1990). Triangulating data. In *Researching Social Gerontology*, Peace, S. (Ed.), pp.115–28. Sage Publications Ltd, London.

Kelly, J.R. (1972). Work and leisure: a simplified paradigm. *Journal of Leisure Research*, **4(1)**, 50–62.

Kelly, J.R. (1990). Leisure and aging: a second agenda. *Society and Leisure*, **13(1)**, 145–67.

King's Fund (1988). *Promoting Health Among Elderly People: A Statement from a Working Group*. King's Fund, London.

King's Fund (1992). *Focus on Carers*. King's Fund, London.

Kirkpatrick, M. (1989). Middle age and the lesbian experience. *Women's Studies Quarterly*, **17(1/2)**, 87–9.

Kuypers, J. and Bengtson, V. (1990). Towards understanding health in older families impacted by catastrophic illness. In *Family Relationships in Later Life*, second edition, Brubaker, T. (Ed.). Sage Publications Inc., Newbury Park, CA.

Lambert, P. and Dolan, J. (1986). *Ethnic Elderly of Derby*. Derby CRE, Derbyshire Social Services and Derbyshire College of Higher Education, Derby.

Land, H. and Rose, H. (1985). Compulsory altruism for some or an altruistic society for all? In *In Defence of Welfare*, Bean, P. *et al.* (Eds), pp.74–96. Tavistock, London.

Laslett, P. (1989). *A Fresh Map of Life: The Emergence of the Third Age*. George Weidenfeld & Nicholson Limited, London.

Lawton, M.P. (1980). *Environment and Aging*. Brooks/Cole, Monterey.

Lawton, M.P. (1983). Environment and other determinants of well-being in older people. *The Gerontologist*, **23(4)**, 349–57.

Lawton, M.P. and Nahemow, L. (1973). Ecology and the ageing process. In *The Psychology of Adult Development and Ageing*, Eisdorfer, C. and Lawton, M.P. (Eds), pp.619–74. American Psychological Society, Washington DC.

Lazcko, F. and Phillipson, C. (1991). *Changing Work and Retirement*. Open University Press, Milton Keynes.

Leather, P. *et al.* (1985). *Review of Home Improvement Agencies*. Department of the Environment, London.

Levin, E. *et al.* (1989). *Families, Services and Confusion in Old Age*. Avebury, Aldershot.

Levinson, D.J. *et al.* (1978). *The Seasons of a Man's Life*. Alfred A. Knopf, New York.

Lewis, J. (1984). *Women in England 1870–1950*. Wheatsheaf, Brighton.
Lewis, J. and Meredith, B. (1988). *Daughters who Care*. Routledge, London.
Lewis, J. and Piachaud, D. (1987). Women and poverty in the twentieth century. In *Women and Poverty in Britain*, Glendinning, C. and Millar, J. (Eds). Wheatsheaf, Brighton.
Lewis, M. (1985). Older women and health: an overview. In *Health Needs of Women As They Age*, Golub, S. and Freedman, R.J. (Eds), pp.1–16. Haworth Press, New York.
Lewis, R.A. (1990). The adult child and older parent. In *Families in Later Life*, second edition, Brubaker, T. (Ed.), pp.68–87. Sage Publications Inc., Newbury Park, CA.
Liddington, J. (1986). One in four: who cares? Education and older adults. In *Adult Education and the Working Class: Education for the Missing Millions*, Ward, K. and Taylor, R. (Eds), pp.143–57. Croom Helm, London.
Lidz, T. (1976). *The Person—His and Her Development Throughout the Lifecycle*, revised edition. Basic Books, New York.
Lister, R. (1990). Women, economic dependency and citizenship. *Journal of Social Policy*, **19(4)**, 445–67.
Little, J. *et al.* (1988). *Women in Cities: Gender & the Urban Environment*. Macmillan Education Ltd, Houndmills.
Llewelyn, S. and Osborne, K. (1990). *Women's Lives*. Routledge, London.
Lodge, B. (1988). *Handbook of Mental Disorders in Old Age*. Open University Press, Milton Keynes.
Long, J. (1989). A part to play: men experiencing leisure through retirement. In *Becoming and Being Old: Sociological Approaches to Later Life*, Bytheway, B. *et al* (Eds), pp.55–71. Sage Publications Ltd, London.
Long, J. and Wimbush, E. (1979). *Leisure and the Over 50s*. The Sports Council and Social Science Research Council, London.
Long, J. and Wimbush, E. (1985). *Continuity and Change: Leisure Around Retirement*. The Sports Council and Economic and Social Research Council, London.
Lopata, H. (1973). *Widowhood in an American City*. Schenkman, Cambridge, MA.
Lopata, H. (1980). The widowed family member. In *Transitions of Aging*, Datan N. and Lohmann, N. (Eds), pp.93–118. Academic Press Inc., San Diego, CA.
Lowry, S. (1991). *Housing and Health*. British Medical Journal, London.
Luker, K. and Perkins, E. (1987). The elderly at home: service needs and provisions. *Journal of the Royal College of General Practitioners*, **37**, 248–50.
MacDonald, B. and Rich, C. (1984). *Look Me In The Eye: Old Women, Aging and Agism*. Spinsters Book Company, San Francisco, CA.
MacKenzie, S. (1988). Balancing our space and time: the impact of women's organization on the British city, 1920–1980. In *Women in Cities*, Little, J. *et al.* (Eds), pp.41–60. Macmillan Education Ltd, Basingstoke.

Mackintosh, S. *et al*, (1990). *Housing in Later Life: The Housing Finance Implications of an Ageing Society*. SAUS, University of Bristol, Bristol.

MacLean, M. and Groves, D. (Eds) (1991). *Women's Issues in Social Policy*. Routledge, London.

Macreadie, C. (1991). *Elder Abuse: An Exploratory Study*. Age Concern Institute of Gerontology, London.

Maitland, N. (1991). Correspondence with Nan Maitland, Bexley Home Share Scheme, London Borough of Bexley.

Major, J. (1992). *Good Housekeeping*, June.

Manton, K.G. (1982). Changing concepts of morbidity and mortality in the elderly population. *Milbank Memorial Fund Quarterly/Health and Society*, **60(2)**, 183–244.

Marcus, A.C. and Seeman, T.E. (1981). Sex differences in reports of illness and disability: a preliminary test of the 'fixed role obligations' hypothesis. *Journal of Health and Social Behaviour*, **22**, 174–82.

Markson, E. (Ed.) (1988). *Older Women: Issues and Prospects*. Lexington Books, Lexington, MA.

Marris, P. (1974). *Loss and Change*. Routledge, London.

Martin, B. (1990). The cultural construction of ageing. In *Aspects of Ageing*, Social Policy Paper No. 3, Bury, M. and Macnicol, J. (Eds), pp.53–81. Department of Social Policy and Social Science, Royal Holloway and Bedford New College, London.

Martin, J. and Roberts C. (1984). *Women and Employment: A Lifetime Perspective*. HMSO, London.

Martin, J. *et al.* (1988). *The Prevalence of Disability Among Adults: Report 1*. HMSO, London.

Marwick, A. (1982). Women's fightback on the home front. *The Times Higher Education Supplement*, 10.9.82, 11–12.

Mason, J. (1987a). *Gender Inequality in Long-term Marriages*, unpublished PhD thesis. University of Kent, Canterbury.

Mason, J. (1987b). A bed of roses? Women, marriage and inequality in later life. In *Women and the Life Cycle: Transitions and Turning Points*, Allat, P. *et al.* (Eds), pp.90–115. Macmillan, London.

Mason, J. (1988a). Married women, ageing and leisure: a sociological contribution. In *Positive Approaches to Ageing: Leisure and Lifestyle in Later Life*, Bernard, M. (Ed.), pp.30–6. The Beth Johnson Foundation in association with the Centre for Social Gerontology, University of Keele, Keele.

Mason, J. (1988b). 'No peace for the wicked': older married women and leisure. In *Relative Freedoms: Women and Leisure*, Wimbush, E. and Talbot, M. (Eds), pp.75–85. Open University Press, Milton Keynes.

Matheson, J. (1990). *Voluntary Work*, GHS No. 17, Supplement A. OPCS, London.

Matrix (Eds) (1984). *Making Space: Women and the Man Made Environment*. Pluto Press, London.

Matthews, S. (1979). *The Social World of Old Women*. Sage Publications Inc., San Diego, CA.

Matthews, S. (1986). *Friendships Through the Life Course, Oral*

Biographies in Old Age. Sage Publications Inc., San Diego, CA.
Mays, N. and Donaldson, L. (1981). *Feasibility Study of the Health and Social Needs of Elderly Asians.* University of Leicester, Department of Community Health, Leicester.
McCalman, J.A. (1990). *The Forgotten People.* King's Fund Centre, London.
McCollum, A. (1990). *The Trauma of Moving.* Sage Publications Inc., San Diego, CA.
McDaniel, S.A. (1989). Women and aging: A sociological perspective. In *Women As They Age: Challenge, Opportunity and Triumph*, Garner, J.D. and Mercer, S.O. (Eds), pp.47–67. Haworth Press, New York.
McDowell, L. (1983). City and home: urban housing and the sexual division of space. In *Sexual Divisions: Patterns and Processes*, Evans, M. and Ungerson, C. (Eds), pp.142–63. Tavistock, London.
McDowell, L. and Pringle, R. (1992). *Defining Women—Social Institutions and Gender Divisions.* Polity Press in association with the Open University, Cambridge.
McEwen, E. (Ed.) (1990). *Age: The Unrecognised Discrimination.* Age Concern England, London.
McFarlane, B. (1984). Homes fit for heroines: housing in the Twenties. In *Making Space: Women and the Man Made Environment*, Matrix (Eds), pp.26–36. Pluto Press, London.
McIntosh, S. (1981). Leisure studies and women. In *Leisure and Social Control*, Tomlinson, A. (Ed), pp.93–112. Brighton Polytechnic, Brighton.
McKinlay, J.B. *et al.* (1989). A review of the evidence concerning the impact of medical measures on recent mortality and morbidity in the United States. *International Journal of Health Services*, **19(2)**, 181–208.
McNair, S. (1984). *Education and Older People*, Pre-Retirement Association Unit News, 7, December. Pre-Retirement Association, Guildford.
Meade, K. (1986). *Challenging the Myths—A Review of Pensioners' Health Courses and Talks.* Age Well, London.
Meade, K. (1987). *Helping Yourself to Health—Health Courses for Older People: A 'How To' Guide.* Pensioners' Link/Health Education Council, London.
Middleton, L. (1987). *So Much for So Few: A View of Sheltered Housing*, The Institute of Human Ageing, occasional papers 3. Institute of Human Ageing, University of Liverpool, Liverpool.
Midwinter, E. (1985). *The Wage of Retirement: The Case for a New Pensions Policy.* Centre for Policy on Ageing, London.
Midwinter, E. (1990). Your country doesn't need you!: age discrimination and voluntary service. In *Age: the Unrecognized Discrimination*, McEwen, E. (Ed.), pp.97–106. Age Concern England, London.
Midwinter, E. (1991a). *The British Gas Report on Attitudes to Ageing 1991.* Burson-Martstellar, London.
Midwinter, E. (1991b). *Out of Focus—The Press and Broadcasting.* Centre for Policy on Ageing, London.

Midwinter, E. (1992). *Leisure: New Opportunities in the Third Age*, Research Paper no. 4. The Carnegie United Kingdom Trust, Dunfermline.

Millar, J. and Glendinning, C. (1989). Gender and poverty. *Journal of Social Policy*, **18(3)**, 363–81.

Mills, R. (1976). Recreational choice: a review. In *Planning for Leisure*, pp.49–56. PTRC Summer Annual Meeting, University of Warwick, Warwick.

Ministry of Health (1962). *A Hospital Plan for England and Wales*, Cmnd. 1604. HMSO, London.

Mitchell, J. and Oakley, A. (Eds) (1986). *What Is Feminism?* Blackwell Publishers, Oxford.

Morgan, K. *et al.* (1987). Mental health and psychological well-being among the old and very old living at home. *British Journal of Psychiatry*, **150**, 801–7.

Morris, J. (1991). *Pride Against Prejudice: Transforming Attitudes to Disability*. Women's Press, London.

Morris, J. (1992). 'Us' and 'Them'? Feminist research, community care and disability. *Critical Social Policy*, **33(Winter 1991/92)**.

Moss, S. and Moss, M. (1989). The impact of the death of an elderly sibling. *American Behavioural Scientist*, **33(1)**, 94–106.

Mullins, C. (1990). *Famine Among Plenty*. Centre for the Analysis of Social Policy, University of Bath.

Murphy, E. (1982). Social origins of depression in old age. *British Journal of Psychiatry*, **141**, 135–42.

Murphy, E. (1988). Prevention of depression and suicide. In *Mental Health Problems in Old Age*, Gearing, B. *et al.* (Eds), pp.67–73. John Wiley and Sons Ltd, Chichester.

Murray, C. (Ed.) (1998). *The Emerging British Underclass*. IEA Health and Welfare Unit, London.

Nathanson, C.A. (1975). Illness and the feminine role: a theoretical review. *Social Science and Medicine*, **9**, 57–62.

Nathanson, C.A. (1977). Sex, illness and medical care: a review of data, theory and method. *Social Science and Medicine*, **11(1)**, 13–25.

National Institute for Social Work (1988). *Residential Care: A Positive Choice. Report of the Wagner Committee into Residential Care*. HMSO, London.

Nestle, J. (1988). *Restricted Country*. Sheba Feminist Publishers, London.

Neugarten, B.L. (1974). Age groups in American society and the rise of the Young-Old. *Annals of the Association of American Political and Social Sciences*, **41(5)**, 187–98.

Neugarten, B.L. (1975). The future of the Young-Old. *The Gerontologist*, **15(1:2)**, 4–9.

Nicholson, J. (1984). *Men and Women: How Different Are They?* Oxford University Press, Oxford.

Nield, S. and Pearson, R. (1992). *Women Like Us*. Women's Press, London.

Nissel, M. and Bonnerjea, L. (1982). *Family Care of the Elderly: Who Pays?* Policy Studies Institute, London.

Norman, A. (1985). *Triple Jeopardy: Growing Old in a Second Homeland*. Centre for Policy on Ageing, London.

Nottage, A. (1991). Gender agenda. *Social Work Today*, **16.5.91**, 12–13.

Oakley, A. (1976). *Women's Work: The Housewife, Past and Present*. Vintage Books, New York.

Oakley, A. (1981). Interviewing women: a contradiction in terms? In *Doing Feminist Research*, Roberts, H. (Ed.), pp.30–61. Routledge, London.

Oakley, A. (1984). *Taking It Like a Woman*. Jonathan Cape Ltd, London.

Oakley, A. (1986). *Telling the Truth About Jerusalem*. Blackwell Publishers, Oxford.

O'Bryant, S. (1983). The subjective value of 'home' to older homeowners. *Journal of Housing and the Elderly*, **1(1)**, 29.

O'Connor, G. (1988). *Back to Work*. Macdonald Optima, London.

Office of Health Economics (1990). *Osteoporosis and the Risk of Fracture*. OHE, London.

Office of Population Censuses and Surveys (1983a). *Fertility Report from the 1971 Census*. HMSO, London.

Office of Population Censuses and Surveys (1983b). *General Household Survey, 1981*. HMSO, London.

Office of Population Censuses and Surveys (1985). *General Household Survey, 1983*. HMSO, London.

Office of Population Censuses and Surveys (1987a). *General Household Survey, 1985*. HMSO, London.

Office of Population Censuses and Surveys (1987b). *Mortality Statistics, 1985 England and Wales*, Series DH2, No. 12. HMSO, London.

Office of Population Censuses and Surveys (1987c). *Population Projections*, Series PP2, No. 16. HMSO, London.

Office of Population Censuses and Surveys (1989a). *General Household Survey, 1986*. HMSO, London.

Office of Population Censuses and Surveys (1989b). *General Household Survey, 1987*. HMSO, London.

Office of Population Censuses (1990a). *Population Trends 61*. HMSO, London.

Office of Population Censuses and Surveys (1990b). *Marriage Series*, FM2 No. 15. HMSO, London.

Office of Population Censuses and Surveys (1990c). *Mortality Statistics, 1987, England and Wales*, DH1 No. 20. HMSO, London.

Office of Population Censuses and Surveys (1990d). *General Household Survey, 1988*. HMSO, London.

O'Laughlin, K. (1988). The final challenge: facing death. In *Older Women: Issues and Prospects*, Markson, E. (Ed.), pp.275–96. Lexington Books, Lexington, MA.

Oldman, C. (1990). *Moving in Old Age: New Directions in Housing Policies*. Social Policy Research Unit, University of York. HMSO, London.

Oliver, M. (1990). *The Politics of Disablement*. Macmillan, London.

Olsen, T. (1980). *Tell Me a Riddle*. Virago Press, London.

Oppenheim, C.   (1990).   *Poverty: The Facts*. Child Poverty Action Group, London.

O'Reilly, D.   (1988).   *Concessionary Fare Schemes in Great Britain in 1988*. Transport and Road Research Laboratory, Crowthorne.

Oxley, P.R.   (1989).   *The Mobility of Disabled People*. Transport and Road Research Laboratory, Crowthorne.

Oxley, P.R. and Benwell, J.   (1989).   *The Use of Buses in Sheffield by Elderly and Handicapped People*. Transport and Road Research Laboratory, Crowthorne.

Pahl, J.   (1989).   *Money and Marriage*. Macmillan, London.

Parker, S.   (1972).   *The Future of Work and Leisure*. Paladin, London.

Parker, S.   (1976).   *The Sociology of Leisure*. Allen & Unwin, London.

Parker, S.   (1980).   *Older Workers and Retirement*. HMSO, London.

Parker, S.   (1983).   *Leisure and Work*. Allen & Unwin, London.

Parker, S.   (1985).   Older women and leisure. In *Leisure and the Elderly in London*, Papers in Leisure Studies, No. 11, Parker, S. (Ed.), pp.18–22. Polytechnic of North London, London.

Patai, D.   (1991).   US academics and Third World women: is ethical research possible? In *Women's Words—The Femininist Practice of Oral History*, Berger Gluck, S. and Patai, D. (Eds), pp.137–53. Routledge, Chapman and Hall Inc., New York, NY.

Peace, S.   (1986).   The forgotten female: social policy and older women. In *Ageing and Social Policy: A Critical Assessment*, Phillipson, C. and Walker, A. (Eds), pp.61–86. Gower Publishing Group Ltd, Aldershot.

Peace, S.   (1987).   Residential accommodation for dependant elderly People in Britain. *Space, Population, Societies*, **1**, 271–80.

Peace, S.   (1988).   Living environments for the elderly: promoting the 'right' institutional environment. In *The Ageing Population: Burden or Challenge?*, Wells, N. and Freer, C. (Eds), pp.217–34. Macmillan Press, London.

Peace, S. (Ed.)   (1990).   *Researching Social Gerontology*. Sage Publications Ltd, London.

Peace, S. and Nusberg, C.   (1984).   *Shared Living: A Viable Alternative for the Elderly?* International Federation on Aging, Washington DC.

Pearson, M.   (1991).   Care of black and ethnic minority elders. In *Nursing Elderly People*, second edition, Redfern, S.J. (Ed), pp.437–47. Churchill Livingstone, Edinburgh.

Percy, K.   (1990).   Opinions, facts and hypotheses: older adults and participation in learning activities in the United Kingdom. In *Ageing, Education and Society*, Glendenning, F. and Percy, K. (Eds), pp.24–46. Association for Educational Gerontology, Keele.

Peterson, D.A.   (1983).   *Facilitating Education for Older Learners*. Jossey-Bass Inc. Publishers, San Francisco, CA.

Phillips, A.   (1987).   *Divided Loyalties: Dilemmas of Sex and Class*. Virago Press, London.

Phillips, D.L. and Segal, B.E.   (1969).   Sexual symptoms and psychiatric symptoms. *American Sociological Review*, **34**, 58–72.

Phillipson, C.   (1982).   *Capitalism and the Construction of Old Age*. Macmillan, London.

Phillipson, C. (1990). Training and education for paid carers: a critical commentary. In *Ageing, Education and Society*, Glendenning, F. and Percy, K. (Eds), pp.157–63. Association for Educational Gerontology, Keele.

Phillipson, C. (1991). Inter-generational relations: conflict or consensus in the twentieth century. *Policy and Politics*, 19(1), 27–36.

Phillipson, C. and Strang, P. (1986). *Training and Education for an Ageing Society*. Health Education Council in association with the Department of Adult and Continuing Education, University of Keele, Keele.

Phillipson, C. and Walker, A. (1986). *Ageing and Social Policy: A Critical Assessment*. Gower Publishing Group Ltd, Aldershot.

Phillipson, C. and Walker A. (1987). The case for a critical gerontology. In *Social Gerontology: New Directions*, di Gregorio, S. (Ed.), pp.1–18. Croom Helm, London.

Piachaud, D. (1987) Problems in the definition and measurement of poverty. *Journal of Social Policy*, 16(2), 147–64.

Pickup, L. (1988). Hard to get around: a study of women's travel mobility. In *Women in Cities: Gender and the Urban Environment*, Little, J. *et al.* (Eds), pp.98–116. Macmillan Education Ltd, Houndmills.

Pitkeathley, J. (1989). *It's My Duty Isn't It?* Souvenir Press, London.

Pitkeathley, J. (1991). The carers' viewpoint. In *Disability and Social Policy*, Dalley, G. (Ed), pp.203–4. Policy Studies Institute, London.

Plant, R. (1985). The very idea of a welfare state. In *In Defence of Welfare*, Bean, P. *et al.* (Eds), pp.3–30. Tavistock, London.

Pritchard, J. (1992). *The Abuse of Elderly People—A Handbook for Professionals*. Jessica Kingsley, London.

Pulling, J. (1987). *The Caring Trap*. Women's Press, London.

Qureshi, B. (1991). Traditions of ethnic minority groups. In *Multicultural Health Care and Rehabilitation*, Squires, A. (Ed.), pp.59–68. Edward Arnold & Age Concern England, London.

Qureshi, H. and Walker, A. (1989). *The Caring Relationship*. Macmillan, London.

Ramazanoglu, C. (1989). *Feminism and the Contradictions of Oppression*. Routledge, London.

Raphael, S. and Robinson, M. (1984). The older lesbian: love relationships and friendship. In *Women-identified Women*, Darty, T. and Potter, S. (Eds), pp.67–92. Mayfield Publishing Co., Mountain View, CA.

Rapoport, R. and Rapoport R.N. (1975). *Leisure and the Family Life Cycle*. Routledge and Kegan Paul, London.

Reddin, M. and Pilch, M. (1985). *Can We Afford Our Future?* Age Concern England, London.

Redfoot, D.L. and Back, K.W. (1988). The perceptual presence of the life course. *International Journal of Aging and Human Development*, 27(3), 155–71.

Rees, C. (1991). *Social Workers, Old Women and Female Carers*, Social Work Monographs. University of East Anglia, Norwich.

Reinharz, S. (1986). Friends or foes: gerontological and feminist theory. *Women's Studies International Forum*, 9(5), 503–14.

Reinharz, S. (1989). Feminism and anti-ageism: emergent connections. In *Health and Economic Status of Older Women*, Herzog, R.A. *et al.* (Eds), pp.24–32. Baywood Publishing Company Inc., New York.

Resource Information Service (1988). *Women's Housing Handbook*. Resource Information Service, London.

Roberto, K. (1990). Grandparent and grandchild relationships. In *Families in Later Life*, second edition, Brubaker, T. (Ed.), pp.100–12. Sage Publications Inc., San Diego, CA.

Roberts, E. (1988). *Women's Work 1840–1940*. Macmillan, London.

Roberts, H. (1985). *The Patient Patients*. Pandora Press, London.

Roberts, H. (1992). Answering back: the role of respondents in women's health research. In *Women's Health Matters*, Roberts, H. (Ed.), pp.176–92. Routledge, London.

Roberts, K. (1970). *Leisure*. Longman Group UK Ltd, Harlow.

Robertson, J.F. (1976). Significance of grandparents: perceptions of young adult grandchildren. *The Gerontologist*, **16(2)**, 137–40.

Rodeheaver, D. (1987). When old age became a problem, women were left behind. *The Gerontologist*, **271(6)**, 741–6.

Rodgers, H.B. (1967). *Pilot National Recreation Survey*. British Travel Authority and the University of Keele, Keele.

Roos, N.P. and Shapiro, E. (1981). The Manitoba longitudinal study on ageing: preliminary findings on health care utilization by the elderly. *Medical Care*, **XIX(6)**, 644–57.

Rosenthal, C. (1985). Kin-keeping in the familial division of labour. *Journal of Marriage and the Family*, **47(4)**, 965–74.

Rosser, C. and Harris, C. (1965). *The Family in Social Change*. Routledge, London.

Rossi, A. (1969). Sex equality: the beginning of ideology. In *Masculine/ Feminine*, Roszak, B. and Roszak, T. (Eds), pp.173–86. Harper & Row, New York.

Rowles, G.D. (1983). Place and personal identity in old age: observations from Appalachia. *Journal of Environmental Psychology*, **3(2)**, 299–313.

Royal College of General Practitioners/Office of Population Censuses and Surveys and the Department of Health and Social Security (1986). *Morbidity Statistics from General Practice, 3rd National Study 1981/2*. HMSO, London.

Sagir, M. and Robins, E. (1973). *Male and Female Homosexuality*. Wilkins and Wilkins, Baltimore, ML.

Saifullah Khan, V. (1979). *Minority Families in Britain: Support and Stress. Studies in Ethnicity*. Macmillan, London.

Sang, B. (1984). Lesbian relationships: a struggle toward partner equality. In *Women-identified Women*, Potter, S. and Darty, T. (Eds), pp.51–66. Mayfield Publishing Co., Mountain View, CA.

⁎ Sargant, N. (1991). *Learning and Leisure*. NIACE, Leicester.

Savo, C. (1984). *Self-care and Self-help Programmes for Older Adults in the United States*. Health Education Council in association with the Department of Adult and Continuing Education, University of Keele, Keele.

Schneider, B. (1984). Peril and promise: lesbians' workplace participation. In *Women-identified Women*, Potter, S. and Darty, T. (Eds), pp.211–30. Mayfield Publishing Co., Mountain View, CA.

Schuller, T. and Young, M. (1991). *Life After Work—The Arrival of the Ageless Society*. Harper and Collins, London.

Scott, G. (1990). Factors influencing the economic vulnerability of older women. In *UN Division for the Advancement of Women, Expert Group Meeting on Vulnerable Women*. UN, Vienna.

Scott, J.P. (1990). Sibling interaction in later life. In *Families in Later Life*, second edition, Brubaker, T. (Ed.), pp.86–99. Sage Publishing Inc., San Diego, CA.

Shanas, E. *et al.* (1965). *Old People in Three Industrial Societies*. Routledge and Kegan Paul, London.

Shapiro, J. (Ed.) (1989). *Ourselves Growing Older: Women Ageing with Knowledge and Power*. Fontana, London.

✳ Shea, P. (1990). The later years of lifelong learning. In *Ageing, Education and Society*, Glendenning, F. and Percy K. (Eds), pp.63–81. Association for Educational Gerontology, Keele.

Shearer, A. (1982). *Living Independently*. Centre on Environment for the Handicapped and King Edward's Hospital Fund for London, London.

Sheffield City Council (1986). *Trapped at Home: The Human Cost of Rising Bus Fares*. Sheffield Campaign Unit, Sheffield.

Sidell, M. (1991). *Gender Differences in the Health of Older People*, Research report. Department of Health and Social Welfare, Open University, Milton Keynes.

Sidell, M. (1992). The relationship of elderly women to their doctors. In *Health Care for Older Women*, George J. and Ebrahim, S. (Eds), pp.179–96. Oxford University Press, Oxford.

Sillitoe, K.K. (1969). *Planning for Leisure*. HMSO, London.

Simenon, G. (1972). *The Cat*. Ninth Omnibus Edition. Penguin, London.

Sinclair, I. (1988). Client reviews: the elderly. In *Residential Care: The Research Reviewed*, Sinclair, I. (Ed.), pp.241–92. HMSO, London.

Sixsmith, A. (1986). Independence and home in later life. In *Dependency and Interdependency in Old Age*, Phillipson, C. *et al.* (Eds). Croom Helm, London.

Slack, P. and Mulville, F. (1988). *Sweet Adeline: A Journey Through Care*. Macmillan, London.

Smith, K. (1988a). *Housing Agencies for Elderly Owner Occupiers*. SHAC, London.

Smith, K. (1988b). *I'm not Complaining: The Housing Conditions of Elderly Private Tenants*. Kensington and Chelsea Staying Put for the Elderly in association with SHAC, London.

Smith, R. (1992). Osteoporosis. In *Health Care for Older Women*, George J. and Ebrahim, S. (Eds), pp.109–29. Oxford University Press, Oxford.

Social Science and Medicine (1989). Special Issue on Self-care. **29(2)**.

Social Services Inspectorate (1992). *Confronting Elder Abuse*. HMSO, London.

Sontag, S. (1978). The double standard of ageing. In *An Ageing*

Population, Carver, V. and Liddiard, P. (Eds), pp.72–80. Hodder & Stoughton, London.

Squires, A. (Ed.)   (1991).   *Multicultural Health Care and Rehabilitation of Older People*. Edward Arnold and Age Concern England, London.

Stacey, J.   (1991).   Can there be a feminist ethnography? In *Women's Words—The Feminist Practice of Oral History*, Berger Gluck, S. and Patai, D. (Eds), pp.111–19. Routledge, Chapman and Hall Inc., New York, NY.

Stacey, M.   (1989).   Older women and feminism: a note about my experience of the WLM. *Feminist Review*, **31(Spring)**, 140–2.

Stanley, J. (Ed.)   (1990).   *Side by Side: Hackney Older Women Describe Their Lives*. Hackney Older Women's Project, London.

Stanley, L. and Wise, S.   (1983).   *Breaking Out: Feminist Consciousness and Feminist Research*. Routledge and Kegan Paul, London.

Stewart, G. and Stewart, J.   (1991).   *Relieving Poverty: Use of the Social Fund by Social Work Clients and Other Agencies*. Association of Metropolitan Authorities, London.

Stevenson, O.   (1987).   *Women in Old Age: Reflections on Policy and Practice*. School of Social Studies, University of Nottingham, Nottingham.

Straw, J.   (1989).   *Equal Opportunities: The Way Ahead*. Institute of Personnel Management, London.

Stuart, A.F.   (1991).   *Growing Older in Metropolitan Suburbs: Environmental Interaction and Prospects for Retirement*, unpublished Ph.D Thesis, Department of Geography, King's College, London.

Sugarman, L.   (1986).   *Life-Span Development: Conecpts, Theories and Interventions*. Methuen, London.

Summerfield, P.   (1984).   *Women Workers in the Second World War*. Croom Helm, Beckenham.

Szinovacz, M. (Ed.)   (1982).   *Women's Retirement: Policy Implications of Recent Research*. Sage Publications Ltd, London.

Szinovacz, M.   (1988).   Beyond the hearth: older women and retirement. In *Older Women: Issues and Prospects*, Markson, E. (Ed), pp.93–120. Lexington Books, Lexington, MA.

Talbot, M.   (1979).   *Women and Leisure. A State of the Art Review*. The Sports' Council/SSRC Joint Panel on Sport and Leisure Research, London.

Taylor, R.   (1988).   The elderly as members of society: an examination of social differences in an elderly population. In *The Ageing Population: Burden or Challenge?*, Wells, N. and Freer, C. (Eds), pp.105–29. Macmillan Press, London.

Taylor, R. and Ford G.   (1983).   Inequalities in old age: an examination of age, sex and class differences in a sample of community elderly. *Ageing and Society*, **3(2)**, 182–208.

Taylor, R. *et al.*   (1983).   *The Elderly at Risk: A Critical Review of Problems and Progress in Screening and Case-finding*, Research Perspectives No. 6. Age Concern England, London.

Thienhaus, O.L. *et al.*   (1986).   Sexuality and ageing. *Ageing and Society*, **6(1)**, 39–54.

Thompson, J.   (1983).   *Learning Liberation*. Croom Helm, London.

Thompson, L. and Walker, A.J. (1987). Mothers as mediators of intimacy between grandmothers and their young adult granddaughters. *Family Relations*, **36(1)**, 72–7.

Thompson, P. *et al.* (1990). *I Don't Feel Old—The Experience of Later Life*. Oxford University Press, Oxford.

Thomson, D. (1989). The welfare state and generational conflict: winners and losers. In *Workers Versus Pensioners: Intergenerational Justice in an Ageing World*, Johnson, P. *et al.* (Eds), pp.33–56. Manchester University Press in association with the Centre for Economic Policy Research, Manchester.

Tilston, J. and Williams, J. (1992). 'Everyone wants to go to heaven but nobody wants to die.' Screening women over 75—a health promotion approach. In *Health Care for Older Women*, George, J. and Ebrahim, S. (Eds), pp.205–21. Oxford University Press, Oxford.

Timaeus, I. (1986). Family and households of the elderly population. *Ageing and Society*, **6(3)**, 271–94.

Tinker, A. (1989). *An Evaluation of Very Sheltered Housing*. HMSO, London.

Tinker, A. (1992). *Elderly People in Modern Society*, third edition. Longman Group UK Ltd, London.

Tomlinson, A. (1979). Leisure, the family and the woman's role— observations on personal accounts. In *Leisure and Family Diversity*, Leisure Studies Association Conference Papers No. 9, Strelitz, Z. (Ed), pp.10.1–10.21. The Sports Council, London.

Tong, R. (1989). *Feminist Thought: A Comprehensive Introduction*. Unwin Hyman, London.

Townsend, P. (1979). *Poverty in the United Kingdom*. Penguin, Harmondsworth.

Townsend, P. (1981). The structured dependency of the elderly: a creation of social policy in the twentieth century. *Ageing and Society*, **1(1)**, 5–28.

Townsend, P. (1986). Ageism and social policy. In *Ageing and Social Policy: A Critical Assessment*, Phillipson, C. and Walker, A. (Eds), pp.15–44. Gower Publishing Group Ltd, Aldershot.

Townsend, P. (1987). Deprivation. *Journal of Social Policy*, **16(2)**, 125–46.

Townsend, P. and Davidson, N. (Eds) (1986). *Inequalities in Health: The Black Report*. Penguin, Harmondsworth.

Townsend, P. *et al.* (1988). *Health and Deprivation: Inequality and the North*. Croom Helm, London.

Trim, A. (1992). Hospital and community nursing of elderly people from ethnic minority groups. In *Multicultural Health Care and Rehabilitation of Older People*, Squires, A. (Ed.), pp.108–21. Edward Arnold and Age Concern England, London.

Turner, B. and Adams, C. (1983). The sexuality of older women. In *Older Women: Issues and Prospects*, Markson, E. (Ed.), pp.55–72. Lexington Books, Lexington, MA.

Twigg, J. (1991). Time on their hands. *The Times Higher Education Supplement*, 25.10.91, p.25.

Uncovering Lesbian History Publications Group (1986). *For Those Who*

Would Be Sisters: Uncovering Lesbian History. Centre for
Extra-Mural Studies, University of London, London.
Ungerson, C. (1983). Women and caring: skills, tasks and taboos. In
The Public and the Private, Gamarnikov, E. *et al.* (Eds), pp.62–77.
Heinemann, London.
Ungerson, C. (1987). *Policy is Personal: Sex Gender and Informal Care.*
Tavistock, London.
Veal, A.J. (1981). *Sports Centres in Britain: A Review of User Studies.*
Centre for Urban and Regional Studies, University of Birmingham,
Birmingham.
Verbrugge, L.M. (1978). Sex and gender in health and medicine. *Social
Science and Medicine,* 12, 329–33.
Verbrugge, L.M. (1984). Longer life but worsening health? Trends in
health and mortality of middle-aged and older persons. *Milbank
Memorial Fund Quarterly/Health and Society,* 62(3), 475–519.
Verbrugge, L.M. (1989). Gender, aging and health. In *Aging and
Health: Perspectives on Gender, Race, Ethnicity, and Class,* Markides,
K.S. (Ed.), pp.23–78. Sage Publications Inc., Newbury Park, CA.
Vetter, N.J. *et al.* (1986). The measurement of psychological problems
in the elderly in general practice. *International Journal of Geriatric
Psychiatry,* 1, 127–34.
Victor, C. (1987). *Old Age in Modern Society.* Croom Helm, London.
Victor, C. (1991). *Health and Health Care in Later Life.* Open
University Press, Milton Keynes.
Voluntary Housing (1987). Housing for older people. *Voluntary
Housing,* special feature, 19(5), 35–50.
Waerness, K. (1990). Informal and formal care in old age: what is wrong
with the new ideology in Scandinavia today? In *Gender and Caring—
Work and Welfare in Britain and Scandinavia,* Ungerson, C. (Ed.),
pp.110–32. Harvester Wheatsheaf, Hemel Hempstead.
Waldron, I. (1976). Why do women live longer than men? *Journal of
Human Stress,* 2, 2–13.
Waldron, I. (1982). Analysis of causes of sex differences in mortality
and morbidity. In *The Fundamental Connection Between Nature and
Nurture,* Gove, W.R. and Carpenter, G.R. (Eds), pp.69–116.
Lexington Books, Lexington, MA.
Walker, A. (1981). Towards a political economy of old age. *Ageing and
Society,* 1(1), 73–94.
Walker, A. (1982). Dependency and old age. *Social Policy and
Administration,* 16(2), 115–35.
Walker, A. (1987). The poor relation: poverty among older women. In
Women and Poverty in Britain, Glendinning, C. and Millar, J. (Eds),
pp.178–98. Wheatsheaf, Brighton.
Walker, C. (1977). Some variations in marital satisfaction. In *Equalities
and Inequalities in Family Life,* Chester, R. and Peel, J. (Eds),
pp.27–40. Academic Press, London.
Wallen, J. (1979). Physician stereotyping about female health and
illness: a study of patient's sex and the information process during
medical interviews. *Women and Health,* 4, 135–45.
Ward, S. (1990). *The Essential Guide to Pensions: A Worker's
Handbook,* third edition. Pluto Press, London.

Warnes, A. and Law, C. (1985). Elderly population distributions and housing prospects in Britain. *Town Planning Review*, **56(3)**, 292–314.

Wearing, B. and Wearing, S. (1988). 'All in a day's leisure': gender and the concept of leisure. *Leisure Studies*, **7(2)**, 111–23.

Webb, I. (1987). *People Who Care—A Report on Carer Provision in England and Wales*. Co-operative Women's Guild, Watford.

Webb, S. (1989). Old lesbians: out and proud. *Social Work Today*, **20(34)**, 20–1.

Wells, B. (1989). The labour market and young and older workers. *Employment Gazette*, **97(6)**, 319–31.

Wells, N. and Freer, C. (Eds) (1988). *The Ageing Population: Burden or Challenge?* Macmillan, London.

Wenger, G.C. (1983). Loneliness: a problem of measurement. In *Ageing in Modern Society*, Jerrome, D. (Ed.), pp.145–67. Croom Helm, London.

Wenger, G.C. (1984). *The Supportive Network: Coping with Old Age*. Allen & Unwin, London.

Wenger, G.C. (1988). *Old People's Health and Experience of the Caring Services: Accounts from Rural Communities in North Wales*. Liverpool University Press, Liverpool.

Wenger, G.C. (1992a). Bangor longitudinal study of ageing. *Generations Review*, **2(2)**, 6–8.

Wenger, G.C. (1992b). Dependence, independence and reciprocity after eighty. In *Aging, Self and Community*, Gubrium, J., Charmaz, K. (Eds), pp.151–74. JAI Press Inc., Greenwich, CN.

Wheeler, R. (1985). *Don't Move We've Got You Covered*. Institute of Housing, London.

Wheeler, R. (1986). Housing policy and elderly people. In *Ageing and Social Policy*, Phillipson, C. and Walker, A. (Eds), pp.217–36. Gower Publishing Group Ltd, Aldershot.

Whitehead, M. (1988). *The Health Divide*. Penguin, Harmondsworth.

Wicks, M. (1987). *A Future for All: Do We Need a Welfare State?* Family Policy Studies Centre, London.

Wilensky, H.L. (1960). Work, careers and social integration. *International Social Science Journal*, **12(4)**, 543–60.

Willcocks, D. (1986). Residential care. In *Ageing and Social Policy*, Phillipson, C. and Walker, A. (Eds), pp.146–62. Gower Publishing Group Ltd, Aldershot.

Willcocks, D. *et al.* (1982). *The Residential Life of Old People: A Study of 100 Local Authority Homes*. Vol. 1. Research Report No. 12. Survey Research Unit, Polytechnic of North London, London.

Willcocks, D. *et al.* (1987). *Private Lives in Public Places*. Tavistock, London.

Williams, G. (1990). *The Experience of Housing in Retirement*. Avebury, Aldershot.

Wilson, A. (1978). *Finding a Voice: Asian Women in Britain*. Virago Press, London.

Wilson, E. (1977). *Women and the Welfare State*. Tavistock, London.

Wilson, E. (1980). *Only Half Way to Paradise*. Tavistock, London.

Wimbush, E. and Talbot, M. (1988). *Relative Freedoms—Women and Leisure*. Open University Press, Milton Keynes.

Winn, L. (Ed.)   (1990).   *Power to the People: The Key to Responsive Services in Health and Social Care*. King's Fund, London.

Witherspoon, S.   (1988).   A woman's work. In *British Social Attitudes: The 5th Report. Social and Community Planning Research*, Jowell, R. *et al.* (Eds), pp.175–200. Gower Publishing Group Ltd, Aldershot.

Women's Design Service   (1991).   *Designing Housing For Older Women*. Women's Design Service, London.

Wood, R.   (1991).   Care of disabled people. In *Disability and Social Policy*, Dalley, G. (Ed.)., pp.199–202. PSI, London.

Wright, F.   (1986).   *Left to Care Alone*. Gower, London.

Young, M. and Willmott, P.   (1973).   *The Symmetrical Family*. Routledge, London.

Zimmeck, M.   (1986).   Jobs for the girls. In *Unequal Opportunities: Women's Employment in England 1800–1918*, John, A.V. (Ed.), pp.153–77. Blackwell Publishers, Oxford.

Index